£22.99

Sociology as Ap
Nursing and Hea

D0549952

For Baillière Tindall:

Publishing manager: Jacqueline Curthoys
Project manager: Ewan Halley
Development editor: Karen Gilmour
Project controller: Derek Robertson
Marketing manager: Hilary Brown

SOCIOLOGY
as Applied to Nursing and Health Care

Edited by

Mary Birchenall MA BA(Hons) RN CertEd RNT
Senior Nursing Lecturer, University of Leeds, Leeds, UK

Peter Birchenall PhD MA RN DN RNT
Professor of Health Studies,
University of Lincolnshire and Humberside, Lincoln, UK

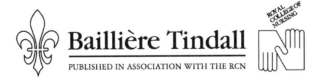

Baillière Tindall

PUBLISHED IN ASSOCIATION WITH THE RCN

Edinburgh London New York Oxford Philadelphia St Louis Sydney Toronto

Baillière Tindall
An imprint of Elsevier Science Limited

First published 1998
Reprinted 2000, 2002, 2003

A catalogue record for this book is available from the British Library.

ISBN 0-7020-1932-1

ELSEVIER SCIENCE your source for books,
journals and multimedia
in the health sciences
www.elsevierhealth.com

Printed and bound in China
W/04

The
publisher's
policy is to use
paper manufactured
from sustainable forests

Contents

Contributors

Mary Birchenall MA BA (Hons), RN, Cert Ed, RNT, Senior Nursing Lecturer, University of Leeds.

Peter Birchenall PhD, MA, RN, DN, RNT, Professor of Health Studies, University of Lincolnshire & Humberside.

John Clayton MSc, FIBMS, Senior Lecturer in Health Studies, University of Lincolnshire & Humberside, Lincoln.

Martin Johnson RN, MSc, PhD, Professor of Nursing, Department of Acute and Critical Care Nursing, University of Central Lancashire, Preston.

Ronnie Moore BSc, DPhil, PGCE, Senior Lecturer, Department of Health and Community Studies, Sheffield Hallam University, Sheffield.

Sam Porter RN, Dip N, BSSc, PhD, Lecturer in Sociology, Department of Sociology and Social Policy, The Queen's University of Belfast, Belfast.

Sandra Ryan RGN, BSc, MSc, Lecturer in Nursing, School of Nursing and Midwifery, The Queen's University, Belfast.

About this book

The Structure and Content of this Book

The book is presented in five sections:

Section 1

The first section introduces the language of sociology, the nature of sociological perspectives and identifies the key areas of sociological study which are of particular importance to the work of nurses and other health-care professionals. The everyday understanding of the social world which the nurse brings into the practice arena is challenged. Key social institutions are examined and related to nursing, the family, education and social class. The principal social groups that are common to all people – gender, ethnicity and age – are reviewed and considered in relation to their significance for nursing practice. These topics have been chosen as having the most common interest to nurses in all four branches, and being the attributes frequently held as significant identifiers for individuals.

Issues such as the nature of the family are examined. The dilemma of accepting personal interpretations of taken-for-granted social institutions, such as the family are revealed, as the familiar group, or family, is explored through the eyes of others who have not shared the same upbringing. Questions are then raised as to the significance of this knowledge for nursing, and for patient, client care and comfort. The sociology of education and social class will also be introduced here and similarly linked to nursing practice.

Key sociological perspectives are introduced. Sociological theories provide a foundation for the final chapter of the book, 'Sociological Perspectives in Nursing' in which the nature of nursing knowledge in relation to sociology is discussed. The issues raised in Section 1 represent the foundation knowledge necessary to moving on to Section 2, which examines the ways in which these individual and social characteristics can influence access to and experience of health care.

<table>
<tr><td rowspan="1">Key concepts</td><td>
<ul>
<li>What is sociology?</li>
<li>Critical language</li>
<li>Sociological perspectives</li>
<li>Social institutions – family, education class</li>
<li>Social groups – gender, 'race' and age</li>
</ul>
</td></tr>
</table>

Section 2

Section 2 is entitled 'Inequalities in Health Care' as it has become evident since the creation of the Welfare State and the National Health Service that some groups of people within our society are healthier than others. This leads to the existence of an apparent inequality in the health status and the health-care provisions. The significance of age, gender, social class and ethnicity to health status is discussed. Questions are raised, although not always answered in a definitive way. Take, for example, the various explanations offered as to why inequalities in health exist at all within a welfare state which offers services to all people, irrespective of background, mainly free of charge.

The main and competing explanations for these inequalities are reviewed. As to which is the correct one you will have to examine your own values and insights and decide as to which is the most persuasive. Poverty as an attribute of lifestyle and its impact on health and health care is considered. Linked to this are the ways in which certain groups within society appear to be disadvantaged due to age, gender and ethnicity. Discussion of some social and health policy issues is a necessary background for the work of nurses and other health-care workers.

Section 2 takes the reader into the somewhat more esoteric world of deviance, linking with the previous discussion on inequality. It reflects on the groups in our society who are stigmatised and as such may experience deficits in health care. This section underpins much of Section 3 and informs some of the material in Section 4.

<table>
<tr><td>Key concepts</td><td>
<ul>
<li>Defining poverty – Historical perspectives on poverty – Reinterpretation of poverty – Poverty in Britain – Poverty and health care</li>
<li>Social class and health – The Welfare State – Welfare rights – Citizenship – Universalism – A changing population</li>
<li>Primary and secondary deviance – Labelling – Stigma – Total institutions</li>
</ul>
</td></tr>
</table>

The concluding part of Section 2 considers again the relevance of these concepts for nurses and health-care professionals; especially when, if asked, the majority of such workers would insist that they treat all patients/clients equally.

Section 3

Having laid some foundations of sociology in the preceding two sections, Section 3 moves into the sociology of nursing and health care, and looks afresh at the ways in which we work with people, whether they are colleagues or clients. The emphasis is on relationships between nurses and colleagues and between nurses and patients/clients. Wider aspects of power and professionalism are considered through a review of key sociological studies that have examined the ways in which the 'tasks' of nursing can lack benefit to the client or patient.

A slight move in direction is taken as Section 3 ends with an overview of professionalisation and the significance of changes in working patterns which require the nurse to work in partnership with many other professionals: the multidisciplinary role. A particular emphasis is the mapping of the nurse as professional, the nature of the relationship between the various 'professional' groups allied to medicine, and the linkage between health-care and social-care arenas.

Key concepts

- Breaking the rules
- Becoming a patient
- The unpopular patient
- Institutionalisation
- Whistle blowing

- The doctor–patient relationship
- Rules in nursing
- Power and social control

- Generalism in nursing
- Professionalisation
- Multiskilling
- Multidisciplinary work
- Nursing specialisms in a changing economy of care
- Normalisation

- Training and education of nurses
- Trade Unionism
- Profession or craft?
- Social model v medical model
- Vocationalism v professionalism

Section 4

In Section 4 the scene moves from nursing work to the wider arenas of the politics of health care. This section concentrates on the changing shape of the National Health Service. The National Health Service and Community Care Act (1990) is reviewed and discussed, with some emphasis on the impact of changes such as the inception of the internal market and Trust status.

Section 4 outlines and reviews that part of the 1990 NHS and Community Care Act which focuses on community care, and considers the possible reasons for the emphasis on 'community' occurring at this time. Within this section, new proposals outlined in the Labour Party General Election Manifesto of 1997 and the NHS White Paper published in December 1997 are introduced. The White Paper aims to give the NHS a 'new lease of life' particularly through changes to the internal market and GP fundholding. New concepts such as locality commissioning, local health-improvement programmes and a national institute for clinical effectiveness are among the developments proposed by the government. Section 4 will consider the changing shape of the NHS and the likely outcomes for the future. Also considered are changes to the delivery of primary health care and how this may affect the nursing role over the next decade. This section is concerned with the social changes which have pre-empted these moves in the health-care system and the interpretation of the impact of such major changes on professional and client worlds.

Key concepts			
■ The NHS Act	■ The founding of the NHS	■ Community
■ NHS Trusts	■ NHS reorganisation	■ Informal care
■ GP contracts	■ Purchaser/provider interactions	■ Informal carers
■ The Health of the Nation	■ Privatisation	■ Women as carers
	■ Cinderella services	

Section 5

The final and concluding section synthesises much of what has preceded and promotes understanding of the significance of the theoretical perspectives of sociology to nursing. The changing role of women in society and the corresponding impact on nursing roles make interesting and perhaps controversial reading as the feminist movement in nursing and midwifery is highlighted.

In concluding, Section 5 encourages the development of a personal perspective which can form the basis for positive reflective practice based in knowledge gained through introspection informed by sociological knowledge, nursing theory and personal practice.

How to Use the Book

Before moving into the main part of the text a brief word about the layout is useful. Each chapter provides references and further reading, useful for the student being introduced to sociology. A glossary of key terms (which are highlighted in bold in the text) is provided at the end of the book, but it may also be useful to have recourse to a sociology dictionary, just in case!

Throughout each chapter there is a range of reflection points, discussion questions and case studies. These provide an opportunity to reflect on and debate some significant issues through applying the theories of sociology to practice. You can use these as part of your own reading and reflection or as the basis for further discussion with other students and colleagues in the practice setting.

At the end of each chapter, the suggestions for further reading are provided to guide you towards key texts of interest.

INTRODUCING THE SOCIOLOGY OF HEALTH CARE

Key concepts
- What is sociology?
- Critical language
- Sociological perspectives
- Social institutions – family, education, class
- Social groups – gender, 'race' and age

The first section introduces the language of sociology, the nature of sociological perspectives and identifies the key areas of sociological study which are of particular importance to the work of nurses and other health-care workers. The everyday understanding of the social world which the nurse brings into the practice arena is challenged. Key social institutions are examined and related to nursing, the family, education and social class. The principal social groups that are common to all people – gender, ethnicity or 'race' and age – are reviewed and considered in relation to their significance for nursing practice. These topics have been chosen as having the most common interest to nurses in all four branches, and being the attributes frequently held as significant identifiers for individuals.

Issues such as the nature of the family are examined. The dilemma of leaving personal interpretations of taken-for-granted social institutions, such as the family are revealed, as the familiar group, or family, is explored through the eyes of others who have not shared the same upbringing. Questions are then raised as to the significance of this knowledge for nursing, and for patient, client care and comfort. The sociology of education and social class is also introduced here and similarly linked to nursing practice.

Key sociological perspectives are introduced. Sociological theories provide a foundation for the final chapter of the book, 'Sociological Perspectives in Nursing' in which the nature of nursing knowledge in relation to sociology is discussed. The issues raised in this section represent the foundation knowledge necessary to moving on to Section 2, which examines the ways in which these individual and social characteristics can influence access to and experience of health care.

1 Studying Sociology in Nursing

Mary Birchenall and Peter Birchenall

Key concepts	■ What is sociology?
	■ Critical language
	■ Sociological perspectives
	■ Social institutions – family, education, class
	■ Social groups – gender, 'race' and age

Nursing is complex: as a field of practice it involves many different people. As a consequence, nurses are required to understand not only many medical conditions and nursing procedures, but also the varying interpretations of care experienced by patients, clients and professional colleagues. Additionally, the nurse needs to be able to envision the practicalities of caring as existing within wider frameworks, that range from the individual, to the immediate area of care and even beyond to the wider social world. This social world extends from the local area to national perspectives and ultimately to world-encompassing influences.

As our society widens its cultural horizons to encompass the global aspects of social life evident in twentieth-century Britain, the nature of the client group rapidly changes. This extends the demands on the nurse already made through the internal variations existing in our own 'British' culture. So, if the nurse is to place the patient or client at the centre of care it is necessary to expand personal understandings of social life.

Linked to these changes at an individual level are the organisational changes which seem a constant part of our modern social world; such as the restructuring of the National Health Service (NHS). At a professional level nursing has moved from a dependence for its curriculum on medicine and housekeeping towards the wider theory bases of the health sciences, of which sociology is but one. This text is concerned with those aspects of sociology that underpin the knowledge base and inform the practice of nursing.

Why Study Sociology?

As indicated above, nursing has changed radically over the past few decades, and is moving towards the development of a clearly outlined theory base discreet to itself. Part of this process is the recognition of those areas of existing science which nursing uses in developing its own knowledge (Robinson & Vaughan 1992).

At a more fundamental level the new student of nursing, perhaps regarding sociology as a subject for the first time, may feel that it is reasonable to question the rationale behind the study of sociology in a nursing programme. A brief 'mind exercise' will help provide some clarification. Think for a moment about those occasions when you meet someone for the first time. Ask yourself, What observations do I make? What questions might I ask in order to get to know this person?

It is likely that you would observe most or even all attributes of that person from the following list:

- Male/female
- Dress
- Accent
- Able/disabled
- Young/old
- Ethnic origins
- Attractiveness
- Personal presentation

From your observations of these attributes and perhaps others that you use, some decisions would be made which enable you to place people into an understandable category.

The use of key visible aspects of an individual provides clues which indicate other significant 'truths'. Using the clues given by dress, accent, presentation, occupation and so on, we come to conclusions about someone that are more implicit than explicit. These quiet observations often influence, possible even determine, the ways in which we will approach a person in the future and the regard in which they are held. It is likely that we also transmit this predetermined caricature of a newly met person to others; an awareness that will be returned to in later chapters. Sometimes it is alarming to become aware that we put people into boxes, but if a moment's thought is taken it becomes apparent that this strategy is one of the ways that help us to make sense out of a very complex world.

The claim that each person is individual and unique is commonly made, but in order to avoid having to check out the reality of what seems obvious about each new acquaintance, conceptual short cuts are necessary, and these include categorising people into groups or bands. This strategy helps us save time in a busy world. Perhaps in prehistoric times, these short cuts not only saved time but also saved our lives, as they would have identified those people who were safe, and those who were a threat to our lives. Links to safety exist today, as some aspects of this categorising process can be centred on who as well as what is safe.

These short cuts to knowing someone are as prevalent in nursing as they are in the wider social world. The need to 'know' someone helps the nurse to feel comfortable, to determine the correct approach, and perhaps even to estimate intelligence and compliance. In the same way, the client perceives the nurse as having certain responsibilities, and attributes specific functions to the role of the nurse.

It is evident that at an individual level there is a need to understand the ways in which we make sense out of the social world, so that there can emerge a greater understanding of the nursing world. As will be seen in the remainder of the book, the social nature of the nurse and nursing work demands that such taken-for-granted ideas about what is good or bad, beautiful or not, able or otherwise must be examined as part of the development of individualised care. Each social being uses a categorising process of some kind. Significantly, nurses must examine the social nature of care and the relationships which are established as part of their profession if they are to continue to develop towards independent practice and advanced practice.

Nursing has made tentative advances into the political arena in recent times, having moved most emphatically away from the 'Doctor's Hand-maiden' image towards an independent professional status (Fatchett 1994). The social and cultural changes of the twentieth century prompt the professional and political developments of nurses and other health-care workers to move away from traditional care practices and services towards the complexities of a multidimensional holism.

Holism in Action

When nursing students commence their training and find that they are to take up courses in sociology, psychology, biology, computing and so on as well as nursing they are often bemused. After all they signed up to be nurses, not sociologists. The emergence of multiple strands to nursing education is paralleled by the emergence of holism and holistic care. Nursing has developed a wide understanding of the need to study society as a way of developing further nursing knowledge, practice and expertise.

Both hospital and community care emphasise health as their focus, acknowledging that caring for ill or traumatised people remains important. Whether services have a health or illness emphasis, the nurse is concerned with individual people, families and/or groups of the population. Each individual experiences the world as a social being and when entering into partnership with the health services, cannot suspend their social character. They need to be cared for as whole persons, rather than having parts of their being 'surgically removed', so to speak, and isolated in order to have treatment or care. The whole person requires care and, thus, the concepts within holism provide greater potential progress for the development of nursing knowledge and practice. To achieve this the nurse must address the five dimensions of health: social, physical, intellectual, emotional and spiritual (Beck et al 1988). Other nursing writers such as Roper et al (1996:25) have identified significant factors that influence the activities of daily living and are essential for the delivery of holistic and individualised care. The five factors listed by Roper et al are biological, psychological, sociocultural, environmental and politicoeconomic. The study of sociology is therefore essential to the provision of holistic care and so to the development of nursing.

The social nature of the patient or client is now established as an important element in the provision of care. As a complement to this the social nature of nursing care itself is also recognised, and is worthy of study in itself. Nursing can no longer be considered as a singular subject. Nor can medical conditions/requirements continue to be seen in isolation from other aspects of social life. Holistic nursing care demands an understanding of the sociology of health care. Added to this, as the individual nurse's ability to see the true individuality of each client develops, the nature of and potential for reflective practice expands.

The physical placement of nursing education into Higher Education reinforces the holistic nature of nursing knowledge and complements similar developments in nursing practice. The social nature of nursing work is both necessary and legitimate study for the nurse. Sociology has moved from a peripheral, sometimes overlooked subject area, towards a new significance as a knowledge base which underpins some aspects of 'Nursing Theory'. As the reader of this text will find, nursing theory becomes eminently more understandable if the originating knowledge base is recognised and understood. For this reason, the first section introduces some theoretical concepts that are significant for nursing work.

References

Beck CM, Rawlins RP, Williams SR 1988 Mental health psychiatric nursing: a holistic lifestyle approach, 2nd edn. CV Mosby, St Louis

Fatchett A 1994 Politics, policy and nursing. Baillière Tindall, London

Robinson K, Vaughan B 1992 Knowledge for nursing practice. Butterworth Heinemann, Oxford

Roper N, Logan WL, Tierney AJ 1996 The elements of nursing, 4th edn. Churchill Livingstone, Edinburgh

Sociology and Everyday Life

Mary Birchenall

This chapter reviews some of the descriptions and analyses of the everyday social world. The Family, Education and Social Stratification form the focus for this chapter; they are known as the key social institutions of our society. The concluding section offers some discussion of the relevance of these social institutions to nursing and health care.

Social stratification and social class are addressed in this chapter although it is recognised that it is not wholly accurate to describe class or stratification as a social institution. Set against this is the reality that social stratification has a wide impact at all levels and is a significant factor in the health experience of individuals and is, as such, referred to in many chapters. It is therefore useful to include class within a discussion on the social institutions.

The Social Institutions

A **social institution** is a way of referring to particular social groupings that are common to the majority of people in a society. Weeks (1972) defines a social institution as having:

'[an] historical existence; they are established and constituted, continuing from one generation to the next as they provide the basic social framework within which each generation lives. They are often seen in terms of the social need or function they serve.'
(Weeks 1972:51).

Using this definition of a social institution, it is evident that the family and education are constants in most societies, although their nature may vary over time and place. In British society, the way in which social position is categorised is another notable constant. Notions of class continue to have a function and are influential within 'the basic social framework'.

Family

Perhaps the **family** is the most familiar of the social institutions. This is unsurprising since the word 'family' stems from the word 'familiar', and is intended to refer to something with which we are comfortable, something familiar. In relation to the study of the sociology of the family, this leaves us with some difficulty since the family that each of us is familiar with does seem to have variations. We will consider some of these variations and then identify the underlying similarities which establish the family as a social institution.

**Activity
2.1**

A casual comparison of the nature of individual families can provide an indication of the apparent range of families that exist in this country.

Using your learning group as your sample population, carry out a small-scale survey on the variable nature of the family: make lists of the people in each individual's family, noting:

- the number who live in the same house;
- the number of family members who live within five miles of each other;
- those who live further away and perhaps even in other countries;
- the range of generations there are in each household.

You may think of other questions as you discuss your family structure. Such an interchange will help in making real the range which is represented by the word 'family'.

The supposedly typical family, consisting of two parents, mother and father with two children, is but one example within a range of groupings that can be described as a family.

The typical family unit of mother, father and children referred to above, is known as a *nuclear family*. Some families include, either within the household or close-by, the grandparents, or aunts and uncles; this multigenerational unit is often referred to as an *extended family*. There are a range of *single-parent families* which become established by deliberate choice or accidentally – through the death of a partner or divorce, separation or abandonment. Families in the 'modern' world can reflect heterosexual or monosexual lifestyles. Gay couples have campaigned for the right to foster and adopt children and are slowly emerging as part of the family scene. Single-parent families have increased from 8% of all families in 1973 to 22% in 1993. The nature of these single-parent families remains that of the lone mother; in 1993 20% of all families were lone mothers compared to 2% of all families with dependent children being made up of a lone father (source: Central Statistical Office 1996). The family can include relationships based on genetics (natural parents) and/or the law (step-parents). When taking differences based on culture into account, there is a broadening of the potential variations in the interpretation of individual understandings of family.

Personal experiences of family life, when combined with images portrayed in the visual and written media, can indicate some common elements shared by all families. For example, each family takes responsibility for child care, income, maintaining the household, and ensuring that a secure and comfortable environment exists within the home. These tasks could be shared by key individuals or be carried out by one particular person. The tasks themselves can be achieved to varying standards. In this way the family can be described has having some core functions that may be considered by some writers as essential to the maintenance of society. The significant groups in a society – those that determine the nature of these functions, define the corresponding acceptable standards and identify the individual family roles – are key subjects within some fields of sociology.

The Functions of the Family

We begin the sociology of the family with a historical review as is usual with any consideration of a social institution. Social institutions can be seen to have functions that help in the establishment and formation of their nature. The functional nature may change over time and between places. Box 2.1 lists the traditional functions of the family that are seen as typical of preindustrial society.

These functions of the family were considered central to the reproduction and maintenance of society. Fletcher (1973) in a study entitled 'The Family and Marriage in Britain' divided these functions into essential and non-essential. The essential functions being reproduction, sexual activity, and the provision of a home; the remaining functions on the list being non-essential. As can be surmised from Box 2.1, in preindustrial society

Box 2.1   Functions of the family in preindustrial Britain

- Reproduction and sexual activity
- Economic provision
- A unit of production
- Child care: Socialisation
            Social control
            Education
            Health and welfare
            Religion
- The family creates a link to society

the family dispensed from within itself many of the functions which today are expected to be provided by external institutions sponsored by the State. For example, health care is today a major and specialised enterprise and the family is expected to use that service. A clear example of this change is the monitoring functions of general practitioners (GP) and health visitors in relation to the infant. The family who does not comply with routine health checks is viewed with suspicion.

A major difference that is evident between preindustrial and modern times is the function of the family as a unit of production. In preindustrial society most people obtained their living from the land, and families would work as units in which most age ranges contributed to the household income. This pattern was replicated to some extent as industrialisation emerged. Families could be employed as a working unit, with a differential scale of pay based on the ages and abilities of the family members. As more complex tasks became mechanised, and the work force diminished, changes were necessary. As children were no longer taken to the workplace their care moved into the home (with mother) and eventually to school.

Ultimately, the functions of the family changed, from a unit of production to a unit of consumption. That is, a central function of the modern family is to consume the products and services of industry. Additionally, as the roles of production and child care became separated within the family, the **gender** divisions of responsibility that are familiar in the present day started to emerge. The combined developments of capitalism and technical progress created a socially determined change in the nature of family life. In many ways parental and child roles, as recognised in the present, emerged with the changing employment scene. These changes are significant for the family, but also make an equally important contribution to the orderly maintenance of an industrial society. The emergence of the industrial age cannot be divorced from the changes in family functions. The breadwinner and the homemaker roles are interdependent within both the family and society.

Other changes in the functions of the family centre on the suggestion that the State has taken over responsibility for such areas as education, health and welfare. One proposal is that the family contributes mainly to the primary or first stage of socialisation. Secondary socialisation occurs outside the family through other social institutions. Fletcher (1973) suggests that this change is less radical than is claimed. He maintains that the family retains its central roles, perhaps to an even more extensive degree than in the 'traditional' family, and is supported by the state in carrying out these functions. Far from the functions of the family being eroded they have actually increased and intensified. Certainly, over the last decade the ideas, espoused by Etzioni, of communitarianism – urging a return to earlier values of the family – have been taken up by senior statesmen including the present British Prime Minister Tony Blair. This communitarian movement and the attention given to it by politicians would seem to endorse the idea that the ideal family is a significant component of society (Kelly 1995). Reporting an interview with Etzioni, Kelly comments

> 'Within the space of 24 hours the professor of sociology had spent an hour with Tony Blair, enjoyed dinner with nine Tory MPs and was looking forward to lunch with Paddy Ashdown. . . . Etzioni believes passionately in the family and is alarmed at its precarious state. "Few who advocate equal rights for women favoured a society in which sexual equality would mean that all adults would act like men, who in the past were relatively inattentive to children. Yet this is what has happened."'
> (Kelly 1995:21)

There are a number of developments over the past years that have both highlighted the changing nature of the family and reinforced the functions of the family particularly in relation to child care and social relationships. Two elements are addressed here; first, the changes in the structure of the family, and second, the societal imperative for families to function adequately.

Changes in the Family

The most common approach to reassessing the family is to compare the types of family evident both in the past and today. Box 2.2 provides a listing of some of the most common labels given to the family. As you will remember, the traditional preindustrial family is often described as an *extended* family. That is a family unit extending over at least three generations. The modern family is referred to as a *nuclear* family, that is, the family unit comprises of two generations only: parents and dependant

Box 2.2   Family Models

- Extended family
- Nuclear family
- Symmetrical family
- Lone-parent family
- Cohabitation
- Mono-gender

children. Neither description is adequate to describe the family either in the past or the present. There are many arguments which suggest that caution is required when creating golden memories of the traditional extended family. These cautionary notes range from disputing the existence of the extended family to claims that it is alive and well and living in or near many households in Britain. Ronald Fletcher has already been mentioned as being critical of suggestions that the functions of the family have been eroded. A different and more critical approach is presented by Gillian Dalley (1988) and Glendinning & Millar (1992).

A further characteristic of the family, as described by earlier research such as that by Wilmott & Young (1975), is that the child on reaching adulthood leaves the family home. In more recent times the decrease in employment opportunities for young people limits their opportunities to live independently of their parents. As you will read later in this book, the poor employment situation for young people has contributed to a growth in homelessness in the young adult population. As ideals of the family are transmitted across generations the move from extended to nuclear family life creates an expectation for parents and their adult children that dependence ends at adulthood. Without the economic resources to support living independently of their natal home many young people are rendered homeless. The charity for the homeless, Shelter, reports rapid increases in the numbers of young people living without a roof and in temporary accommodation. A vicious circle seems evident between the need for paid employment to finance personal housing and the social norm of leaving home as a measure of adulthood. The situation just described does of course have variations betweeen the social classes. The extension of education for middle-class children does provide a buffer to some extent. However, as current government policies create real costs for higher education there are likely to be further changes in the homeless population and possibly in the nature of the family. Perhaps after the year 2000 British society will see the return of the extended family as a norm, as a consequence of the economic pressures. Alternatively, the young people who enter the next millennium as adults may modify the nature of the family again with several decades of homeless experiences as the catalyst for change (Table 2.1).

Table 2.1

People in households in the United Kingdom: by gender, age and family type (%), Winter 1994–95

	One person	Couple No dependent children	Couple Dependent children	Lone parent	Other person[1]	All persons (=100%) (millions)
Males						
16–19	6	–	–	–	93	1
20–29	23	19	19	1	38	5
30–44	15	19	58	1	6	6
45–59	13	61	22	1	4	5
60–74	20	77	1	–	2	4
75 and over	35	63	–	–	2	1
Females						
16–19	8	3	2	3	85	1
20–29	17	22	26	13	23	4
30–44	8	18	57	13	4	6
45–59	13	65	12	3	7	5
60–74	35	60	–	–	5	4
75 and over	68	27	–	–	5	2

1 People who were not heads of family unit or dependent children
Note: not all figures add up to 100% due to rounding
Source: Central Statistical Office 1996

Family Roles and Relationships

One important feature remains concerning the family – the nature and expectations of the internal family relationships. The early agrarian extended family is frequently described as an egalitarian unit that supported the wider family network. The position of men and women is reflected as being equal, a notion refuted by critics as idealistic. The post-industrial, working class extended family is described by Wilmott & Young (1969) as being typically multigenerational, with married daughters living with or near the mother. The relationships within the household reflected societal expectations; that is the man was head of the household, making important economic decisions, and the woman ruled the home. The internal home structure is defined as *matriarchal* – ruled by the mother. The balance of power is, however, clearly held by the head of the household, father; an example of *patriarchal* power.

The nuclear family shows the man at the head of household, providing for his wife and children, and receiving domestic services in return. This latter is sometimes referred to as *segregated role relationships*. As a unit the nuclear family seemed to increase in incidence as manufacturing industries grew and demanded a more mobile workforce. Additionally, a geographical removal between the generations occurred, removing daughters from the locality of their mothers once they had married. A continuation study by Wilmott & Young in 1975 suggested that this geographical dispersal of family members contributed to changes in the make-up of the family. As married daughters moved away from the maternal home the dissolution of the extended family occurred with a corresponding growth of the *symmetrical family*. Wilmott & Young (1975) define the symmetrical family as moving towards more egalitarian role sharing; for example, women often take up paid employment and the husband participates in the household chores and child rearing.

Symmetrical relationships are characterised by a joint conjugal role relationship; this is a more evenly balanced role relationship, but one that is heatedly contested as having any reality, an issue we will return to in the next chapter in a discussion of gender roles.

> 'The sociological evidence suggests that only a very small minority of men participate in domestic work on anything like an equal basis. This finding holds regardless of whether wives work outside the home or whether they are full-time houseworkers.'
> (Maynard 1985:140)

Some Consequences of Changing Family Functions

An immediate and direct result of this mobility is the disappearance of support for newly married couples and eventually a diminishment in the physical support possible for elderly parents. Ormerod & Rowthorn (1997:16) suggest that the changing nature of the family – in particular divorce and lone parenting – creates a major burden for the state in providing care for the elderly. They write

> 'The growth of lone-parent families, divorce and family reorganisation is creating many millions of people without close family ties. In the future these trends will impose a huge financial burden on the state, since many of those concerned will be unable to afford professional care as they age.'

The negative images of family violence, child abuse and reports of the dissolution of the family through divorce and out of marriage childbirth are some of the factors that prompt the demand for a return to basic principles and family values. The family remains an important ideal in British society, one that has promoted extensive debate in the Houses of Parliament. Questions in the House, addressed to and by past and present leaders, have focused on the assumed evils of single parenthood. These have been expressed as a need to recall people to the positive values of the traditional family for the protection of society.

Finch & Mason (1993) in their book Negotiating Family Responsibilities, highlight the lack of clarity that exists in our society about intrafamily relationships.

'Thus we can say with some confidence that our survey data show that there is nothing approaching a clear consensus about family responsibilities. In the late 1980s in Britain people apparently were not acknowledging clearly identifiable principles about what kinds of assistance family members should offer each other. There is no evidence of a clear acknowledgement at this public normative level that families should be the first line of support for their members. This is something of a contrast with assumptions made in social policy. Leaving aside the question of what people will actually be prepared to do in practice it seems that, even at this level, relatives cannot be relied upon to acknowledge that they have clear responsibilities.'

(Finch & Mason 1993:21)

Reflection point 2.1

Sociological studies of the negative impact of institutional care have contributed to an image of the family as the centre of social and health care. Community care reinforces the need for the family and early indications are that the caring function of the family from birth to death is being reinforced.

The Family Policy Studies Centre (FPSC) strongly urges governments to carefully consider the impact of government actions on families. In study groups you may consider the consequences for families of Community Care legislation.

Question: 'Could Community Care create changes in the family that are as far reaching as those evident after the mechanisation of industry?'

The family is essential for the successful development of wider ranging community care services. In contrast to this need there seems to be an increase in divorce, greater reporting of abuse and violence towards partners and children. For some writers, such as Laing (1965), the family is responsible for many evils and is a destructive force. Frequently the moral panic expressed at the growth in the number of single parents overshadows the hardships of young unsupported women with one or more children.

The problem family

A major development in the study of the family is the emergence of the deviant or problem family. Leaving aside any problems which families may

Reflection point 2.2

Family facts

Divorce figures in the UK show a small growth rate in comparison to the rest of the European Community (EC) 3.1 per thousand population in the UK against 1.7 EC average

A third of all 1993 marriages in the UK were remarriages

Lone parent households increased to 22% in 1993: 20% lone mothers with 2% lone fathers

32% of all live births occur outside of marriage

Lone parenthood varies amongst ethnic groups: 20% of families from the Black ethnic group are lone parents; families from the Indian ethnic group have the lowest percentage of lone parenthood

Single mothers are younger (25 years on average) than married mothers (30 years on average)

Teenage conception rates are falling but remain above the Health of Nation target set for the year 2000

Cohabiting increased to 23% of all non-married women aged 18–49 years in 1994: there is a trend towards longer periods of cohabitation

Household size has decreased from an average of 2.9 to 2.4 in 1994/95: 27% of all households in 1994/94 are made up of one person

Two main reasons for the increase in lone person households can be identified: an increase in elderly people who often live alone, and a recent upsurge in the number of young men living alone, a trend anticipated to continue

All figures taken from Central Statistical Office (1996)

experience as a consequence of violence, or a lack of income, the 'problem family' is often defined by those in powerful positions as a problem to the state. It is not unusual to read or hear media presentations that report the 'problem' family as a burden on society. This may occur through a reliance on welfare support or a perceived inability of those responsible to 'control' their children: a clear example of a threat to society by the abdication of responsibility for the family function of socialisation.

With the political espousal of communitarianism, the controlling functions of the family can be seen to be to the fore once again. Within this moralistic argument, mothers in particular are reminded of their responsibilities towards their children.

Communitarianism seems to have emerged as a response to the 'moral panic', evident in both America and this country, concerning the collapse of the traditional family. The family as a central pillar of society is re-established through rhetoric based on the 'good old days'. It does seem that the emphasis on patriarchal values in the communitarian movement glosses the struggles and hardship of earlier years, always a danger when looking back through rose tinted glasses.

Activity 2.2	The Price of Family Values?

Heather Joshi writes:

'The price a man pays for parenthood is generally being expected to support his children and their mother. The price a woman pays is that of continuing economic handicap and an increased risk of poverty.'
   (1992:124)

Earlier she asserts:

'Foregoing earnings as a result of parenthood is a price ... paid by women but not by men. ... We would suggest that the caring work of a wife may also help to raise the amount that men are paid.'
   (1992:119)

Discuss in your tutorial groups some reasons as to why feminist writers are concerned with the economic consequences of family roles.

Summary

Despite the negative images the family remains, and alternatives to the family emerge with infrequency, examples being the kibbutzim and the commune. Arguments continue as to whether the biological needs for protection and nurturing of the young imply that the family unit in some form is a natural necessity; others demonstrate vehemently the social construction of the family.

There is no surprise in finding that the family is a changing structure that is not constant and similar for each individual. When cultural differences are added to the picture the family becomes diverse indeed. In turn it is an important social institution which, as we will see later, is central to many aspects of health care. Rooted in idealism as well as history this social institution, which is both familiar and alien in parts, is often understood on the basis of individual experiences. As a social institution its effects on society are wide ranging, emerging from the reproduction of and ordering of society to the determination of individual life chances. The shape of the family has two dimensions, the real experiences of people and the ideal examples which are presented to us through such media as television, newspapers and the expectations set within our cultural norms and values. Dalley (1988:16) writes: 'The nuclear individualistic family is the reality for relatively few, but the model for many.' The social dimensions of the family are many and varied; it is not possible to cover them here. What has been achieved is an introduction to some of the key elements of the many studies that focus on the family enabling the reader to successfully key into these texts.

Education

This section focuses on one of the areas that is given as a function of the family: education. As was recognised above, the state takes a dominant part in the provision of education. The emphasis here is to consider education as part of the socialising processes experienced by all or perhaps, more accurately, almost all members of society. Again the functions of education will plot a pathway through the many possible interpretations of this social institution.

The modern education system is an important part of the socialisation process providing the developing child with a secondary set of experiences beyond the family – secondary socialisation. Three main areas are outlined in relation to the role of education in the maintenance of society: social control, equal opportunities and employment.

Education as Social Control

Society can be seen as an artefact, that is, it is constructed by humankind. The major maintenance of this artefact is carried out through the various processes of socialisation. The family is recognised as the prime provider of primary socialisation, within which the young person internalises the values and norms which permeate his or her immediate culture. Education provides a secondary socialisation process, through which children and young people continue to develop their norms and values, learning the rights and wrongs of behaving in public. This process of socialisation is an important part of **social control**.

The phrase 'social control' sounds as though there are external forces coercing individuals. This would be a very demanding way of creating some form of common understanding of the rules and regulations that we all live by. The internalisation at an early age, of the codes of conduct generally expected, ensures that social control over the everyday aspects of life can exist relatively unnoticed by most people. It is a measure of the success of the various socialising processes that we feel self-motivating and self-determining in large areas of our lives. The education system provides an important foundation in establishing these controls.

Both formal and informal control strategies come in to play to ensure the internalisation of norms and values. Written rules and regulations often contribute to formal control; for example, rules on punctuality, dress code, discipline and timetables usually exist. Control agents such as 'prefects' help in creating a successful process. Informal control forms part of the hidden curriculum, and contributes to the expectations of teachers in relation to ability, gender and so on. The combination of these two aspects, formal and informal control, promotes a conforming adult; that is one who both acts and is restrained from acting in ways appropriate to their specific culture. As we will see in the next section on equal opportunities, these mechanisms of social control, which are essential to the transmission of societal values, assist in the reproduction of social inequality.

Education and Equal Opportunity

The creation of greater equality of opportunity is a major imperative in recent reforms of the British education system. The emergence of the comprehensive school in the 1960s from the divisive tripartite system was an early move to create greater equality. Rather than schools being divided along class lines a large neighbourhood school that provided services for all children would contribute to the breaking down of class barriers. This system has not wholly succeeded. When the educational attainment of young people exiting from comprehensive education is measured, middle class children continue to score higher than working class children. Also, girls have diminished experiences in relation to boys, as do children from ethnic minority groups in relation to 'white' children.

Such results could be used to demonstrate that the comprehensive 'experiment' is a failure. There are many pockets of grammar schools still surviving in Britain and, of course, the public school sector has always been able to select suitable candidates through entrance examination and ability to pay. More recently, the 'independent' schools have emerged, with their own rules and regulations in relation to selection and focus. League tables, based on and showing scholastic success as measured by exam results, are now presented for public scrutiny. The reluctant engagement with the ideals of comprehensive education when combined with the development of the 'league' tables, seems to indicate a major impetus towards a re-emergence of the imbalance evident in the tripartite system.

Educational attainment is often taken as an indication of ability. Results such as those for GCSE and 'A' level, when broken down into class groupings, show that the results are good for the middle classes and poor for the working classes. If all children and young people experience education in the same school, then it could be proposed that this discrepancy in achievement between the classes is a result of ability rather than social class. In a more formal language, the educational system is seen by society at large to represent a **meritocracy**; that is a system in which ability is rewarded – success gains merit. Within a meritocracy all who have ability can and should succeed. If there is a gap between the social classes then this is seen as the result of individual ability, and not of social advantage. One suggestion could be that the social classes represent some sort of natural order. Set against such arguments are those that recognise the significance of primary and secondary socialisation in maintaining the status quo within society, and so constructing the social order in ways that seem natural.

Alison Utley reports in the Times Higher Education Supplement (29 August 1997) on the research of John Knowles who has found that there is a clear link between social class and successfully gaining a university place. Knowles found that 30–50% of pupils from schools in disadvantaged areas continued in education after 16 years whereas the national average is for over 70% of young people to take up post-16 education. It seems that a previous generation's experiences of education can limit the horizons of the young and so perpetuate inequalities. Additionally, the new Labour proposals to introduce tuition fees do seem to reduce opportunities for the disadvantaged groups in society. If advancement in society is linked to education, then any movement that limits equality of opportunity in education contributes to the maintenance of class-based society.

Activity 2.3	The British educational system is classed by some as a meritocracy. To what extent is ability alone a factor in educational success?
	Through discussion with your peers and friends you can identify through personal experiences the various issues that contribute to a successful measurement of ability.

Educational attainment is influenced by a range of experiences which have an impact on measured ability. The key groupings have already been listed: they are social class, '**race**' and **gender**. Each of these three groups are considered at greater length in the next chapter. Here we will consider some of the common denominators which contribute to the lack of equality evident within the educational system.

The Home and the School

One of the earlier studies in schools (Douglas 1969) reported that malnutrition and poor home environments were impeding the progress of otherwise able children. He concluded that the failure of many working class children was due to poverty and in particular to hunger. He saw this situation as a waste of future resources and made some proposals to limit this situation, one of which resulted in 'free school milk' for all children.

Douglas as a medical practitioner clearly saw the links between educational performance and health. There is a direct link to wealth and social class in these findings. It is the child who comes from an economically poor home who is most likely to experience nutritional deprivation and suffer the deficits noted by Douglas. He also recounted that middle class parents were involved and concerned about their child's education, whereas the working class parent rarely visited the school and seemed uninterested in education. The privileged position of professional people to take time out of the main working day to visit the school without loss of earnings, unlike the average factory worker who would lose pay, is omitted in such measurements of interest.

Activity 2.4	Two families:
	    Dominic is the only child of professional parents.
	    Ronald is the only child of 'wageless' parents.
	
	Plot a likely life map for the two, highlighting potential differences in their careers. Is it possible to make these assumptions?
	
	A brief foray into *Social Trends* (Central Statistical Office 1996) will provide evidence that can contribute to a typical life path for two people from different backgrounds.

Education and Language

Much has been written about language style and education. Bernstein (1971) describes the working class use of language as being presented in a shorthand style which leaves many unspoken gaps, requiring the listener to fill in by inference the missing parts of the message. In contrast, the middle class use of language is more elaborate, providing detail and using a reasonable semblance of grammatical structure. These codes are respectively referred to as restricted and elaborated codes of language. The teacher uses an elaborated code within the classroom, which implies that the middle class child hears a familiar language that is alien to the working class child. As the teacher speaks to the whole class in a similar way, he or she may feel that equality in the classroom exists. In reality, the opportunities for new learning are less direct for the working class child, who is hearing what is essentially a new way of speaking.

Other writers in this area include Labov (1973), who argued that the apparently restricted language of poor black children in America was as laden with abstract concepts as the more formal dominant white language. Labov demonstrated that the ability to conceptualise was not diminished by a shorthand language. Further, he suggests that the classroom becomes a hostile environment as a consequence of the teacher attempting to impose his or her language code. Such action silences the child and leads to a detachment from the educational process. These writings encourage us to reflect on the potential for prejudging ability due to accent, dialect and class differences in language. The next section demonstrates the problems inherent in such prejudice.

Pygmalion in the Classroom

Rosenthal & Jacobson (1968) researched the impact of the teacher's pre-conceptions concerning ability on the achievements of individual students. In brief, they interviewed teachers to ascertain which children they considered to be less or more able. The expectations of teachers did seem to reproduce the class divisions outlined above. The researchers then carried out IQ tests on each child. They reported their findings to the teachers, but gave misinformation concerning the abilities of some children. In one example, they told teachers that child x had scored high and child y low, although in truth the results of the test were the reverse. The two researchers returned six months later, re-tested the children, and found that child x showed an increased IQ score and child y's score was lower. The teacher had responded to the bogus information in such a way that the researchers' prophecy was fulfilled. It is interesting that the experiment was able to demonstrate that teachers' expectations of a child's ability have a significant impact on the measured performance of that child. It is likely that a self-fulfilling prophecy is an established part of the hierarchy in society and one which contributes significantly to the maintenance of inequalities. When the league tables for schools are produced the social class divisions can be seen to be reproduced. When reading down such league tables some patterns emerge that do seem to corroborate the difficulties that many schools, situated in poorer areas of the country, have in promoting the merits of their pupils.

Education and Employment

Like the family, there is an expectation that everyone has some experience of the education system. Educational achievements are used by employers and higher education as a means of identifying appropriate candidates. Such performance indicators will have impact on the attitudes of employers with regard to the educational background and therefore individual ability of prospective employees. This section considers the influence of education on employment. It is becoming increasingly difficult for anyone to access nurse training without having gained educational qualifications. As nursing education becomes part of the university sector then further changes can be anticipated in relation to the minimum entry qualifications. Perhaps this aspect of health care will emulate other health-care professions and become an all graduate profession; this is, of course, speculation at this moment in time. So, education as a doorway to the workplace does seem to be a reality. The use of meritocratic results is widespread throughout the employment sector. Writers such as Watts (1985) suggest that the use of educational results are seen to be publicly defensible, are convenient for universities to administrate and, importantly, appear to be socially equitable.

Throughout school life young people are encouraged to achieve so that they can improve their future opportunities. As employment has become less certain it is common for educational qualifications to be used in relatively unskilled employment. Increasing youth unemployment may encourage some young people, who are 'failing' in the school environment, to reject education as being of no intrinsic worth to them, as it is unlikely to prepare them directly for future work. Conversely, if employment is scarce, then the failure to achieve within the educational system is taken on board by out of work young. 'If I'd tried harder at school I wouldn't be in this situation now' is often heard.

The function of the school to maintain the status quo within society is hidden and the consequences rarely made overt. It is perhaps through the impact of education on employment that the full consequences of the function of social control and the recurrence of social inequalities can be seen. The educational system is viewed as a meritocracy which rewards ability irrespective of background. Some research reviewed earlier has demonstrated that prejudgements as to potential ability often limit the successful achievements of working class children. The common use of **credentialism** as the first point of access to employment promotes an imbalance of opportunity in the workplace. These features combine to establish, maintain and justify the social inequalities. These latter can take on the appearance of being within the control of the individual rather than being an imposition as an implicit consequence of social control. The next section extends these thoughts as we turn to consider the issue of social class.

Activity 2.5

Using local and national newspapers look through a range of job adverts. Focus on those jobs which are likely to be aimed at the new starter.

Discuss the possible nature of the job and the relevance of the entry qualifications in the advertisements. You may find the following questions useful.

Are employers using entry requirements for more than making a judgement about the relevance of the educational background of the candidates?

Why may employers ask for educational qualifications for jobs that have not in the past attracted candidates with GCSEs?

Social Class

Reference to social class has been made on several occasions. Weeks (1972) whilst commenting that social class is one of the most widely used concepts in sociology, defines social class as referring to 'categories of individuals or groups based on measures of power, income, wealth, prestige, relationship to the means of production or occupation' (Weeks 1972:44). As a term it is relatively familiar: it is frequently used in newspapers and in television as though an absolute and meaningful idea. There are even references to the current emergence of a classless society; perhaps the notion of inequality of opportunity is less acceptable than this to the majority of people. There exist, however, very real divisions between large groups of people and the implications of such inequalities for health care is a central feature of later discussions.

One problem particular to social class is that it is not a single concept; it is part of a theory of stratification. In this respect the theoretical perspective which influences the writer or reader will have direct impact on the discussion. The divisions and relationships across the theoretical formulations of sociology are introduced in Chapter 4. To pursue theories of stratification further the ideas of key theorists need to be outlined here.

There are two main theorists who have influenced understandings of social class: Marx, and Weber (Box 2.3).

Box 2.3   Two theories of Class

Marx presents a structural theory of class in that he identifies two main groups of people who are placed in opposition to each other through their relative positions in the workplace. (In Marxian terms this would be referred to as being in 'relation to the means of production'.) That is, the worker (proletariat) or the owner (bourgeoisie) are opposed forces created through their positions within the system of production.

Weber echoed the importance of economic factors, but rejected a simple twofold distinction within the framework of employment. He suggested that class also has an effect upon life chances, the opportunities to gain or lose positive experiences and opportunities. He adds the dimension of status to the discussion of class. The idea of life chances in relation to social class is significant in later chapters when we consider the ways in which inequality and health are interrelated.

The concept of '**class**' is a relatively modern term and has particular meaning in the United Kingdom. British history makes constant reference to ways of differentiating between large groups of people and so providing insights as to their relative social status. Memories of the feudal system are currently romanticised through tales of heroic figures such as King Arthur and Robin Hood. But the feudal system ensured that the social order of this country remained static as movement between the levels was almost impossible. The present day monarchy is a remnant of that early system of social stratification. The aristocracy are not represented in any currently used classification system, remaining outside the measures that define the majority of society.

Other countries also use systems of social classification, the most well known being those of 'caste' and 'slavery'. The latter may feel as though it belongs to other periods of time but slavery continues to be evident in many parts of the modern world. The caste system is most commonly associated with India; individuals inherit their caste and movement between castes cannot occur, to the extent that interaction between castes is socially unacceptable.

Many sociological studies include a reference to social class without directly linking it to a particular theory. Perhaps there is an assumption that class, like family, is so familiar to readers that the concept can be described in a more pragmatic way, for example, by focusing on the Registrar General's Classification system (Box 2.4). Class is a significant mode of classification and the most commonly used system of representing the social classes remains the Registrar General's Classification. This system is a hierarchical scale of jobs presented in order according to their relative esteem within society.

Box 2.4

Registrar General's Classification
Examples of occupation

Social Class 1	Professional	Doctor, Lawyer, Dentist
Social Class 2	Managerial	Manager, Nurse, Teacher, Librarian
Social Class 3a	Non-manual & Clerical	Policeman, Sales representative, Clerk
Social Class 3b	Manual & Skilled manual	Electrician, Bus Driver, Cook
Social Class 4	Semi-skilled manual	Postman, Barman, Telephonist
Social Class 5	Unskilled manual	Porter, Cleaner, Labourer

As you examine the list in Box 2.4 there should be no surprises as to those occupations that appear at Social Class 1 and those which appear in Social Class 5. The emphasis on occupation reveals that those who are wealthy without employment are outside of this classification, as indeed are those who are not in employment but are poor. You may be surprised to find nursing in Social Class 2.

What is particularly interesting about the Registrar General's Classification is the reason for its creation. There was a recognition of a seemingly higher incidence of ill-health in the poorer sections of society, and some means of verifying this notion was required. The scale was established so that data about births and deaths in particular could be collated and analysed by social class. The complete scale has an extensive listing of occupations within each category, which is far more elaborate than the small selection in the examples given. Since its inception the scale has been highly criticised, although it remains widely used in government reports and surveys. The Registrar General's Classification is frequently represented as a pyramid, with the base being formed by Social Class 5 and the apex by Social Class 1 (Fig. 2.1).

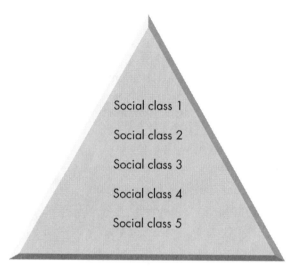

Social class 1

Social class 2

Social class 3

Social class 4

Social class 5

Figure 2.1   **The pyramidal structure of the Registrar General's Classification indicating that the majority of the population is based in the lower social classes**

Such a representation is intended to indicate that the majority of people in society are based in the lower social classes. Changes in the structure of society have emerged, many of which are established through the changing nature of the work place. Due to advances in technology there has been a major shift away from intensive labour on the shop floor. This reduction in unskilled and semi-skilled labour is mirrored by an

Reflection point 2.3

Classification systems that use employment as a key measure have difficulty in categorising people who are not in employment. This includes the unemployed and people in caring roles in the home.

Where do people who have no employment fit in to this shape or those who are homeless, or travellers?

Is it likely that when made visible in the statistics they contribute to re-creating the pyramid shape?

increase in the numbers of administrators and small business men and women. The traditional pyramid of the classes moves to a diamond-like shape, showing the majority of the population as belonging in Social Classes 3a and 3b (Fig. 2.2).

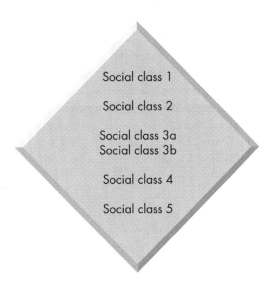

Social class 1

Social class 2

Social class 3a
Social class 3b

Social class 4

Social class 5

Figure 2.2   **A diamond–like structure indicating a reduction in semi– and unskilled labour and the movement of the majority into Social Classes 3a and 3b**

Such a shift in the make-up of society prompts claims of a classless society becoming a reality in the near future. The Marxian term embourgeoisement is used to refer to this merging of the middle and working classes as prosperity and living standards appear to improve.

The flaws in the Registrar General's Classification were recognised in the 1970s by Goldthorpe & Hope (1974) who offered a three-tier representation of the social classes. The basis of the divisions in this scale are the giving and receiving of orders.

- Service Class
  1. Higher grade professionals
  2. Lower grade professionals
- Intermediate Class
  3. Clerical, sales and other service workers
  4. Owners of small businesses, self-employed workers
  5. Lower grade technicians and foremen
- Working Class
  6. Skilled manual workers
  7. Semi-skilled and unskilled workers

Goldthorpe & Hope's scale seems to take into account the changes in occupational structure which have emerged as a result of the growth of administration and increasing numbers of small businesses. The absence of those who are not employed from these classifications underlines the social significance given to employment. In Weber's terms our status or prestige in society is directly linked to our social role which in turn for the majority of people is linked to employment. This is evident to the extent that status in the workplace usually overflows into other areas of life.

However, both Goldthorpe & Hope's classification system and the Registrar General's Classification are based on occupation, a factor that excludes those who cannot be classified according to occupation. In particular, married women, or women living in their parent's home, are invisible within these classifications as they are ascribed a social class through their husband or father. Interestingly, the majority of the population which is classified as skilled non-manual are female; conversely, skilled manual are predominantly male. It may have seemed acceptable at one stage in our social history to ignore the status of women as individuals, referring to them through their husband's or father's status, but this is inappropriate in the present day.

Let us consider for a moment the rationale for focusing on male occupation in determining social class. The arena of paid employment has been regarded as a male preserve until relatively recently. There has been a slow movement towards recognising women as independent members of society, about which there is more to say in Chapter 3. For now, if we recall the function of socialisation in the reproduction of society, we realise that there is a key issue here in relation to the role of women. By subsuming a woman's class within that of her husband's or father's there is an implicit affirmation of the traditional female role being linked to unpaid work. The role of mother may have a high moral value but as an unpaid role it is low in status in relation to such occupations as doctor, teacher or nurse. For some women, the hiding of personal identity within that of any male is an affront to self and dignity. Essentially then, the use of the male occupation, or the 'head of the household', implicitly referring to the man reaffirms the patriarchal nature of power balances within the British social structure.

Discussion questions 2.1

How useful are employment based classification systems in indicating social class?

Would anything significant occur in the hierarchy of these scales if usefulness and necessity directed the structure rather than status?

So far class has been described through two classification systems which enable a structured approach to describing the hierarchy of British society. Significantly, the notions of working class and middle class are understood and used by the majority of people. Newspapers and magazines publish quizzes which purport to place people into their social classes by way of dress, manner, education and attitudes to life. As became evident in the previous section on education, even individual potential for achievement is regarded as being linked to social class. There have been attempts to oppose such classification systems which seem to be based on criteria established through tradition rather than the degree to which a society needs that group of people. Some events from recent social history can help explain this further. Refuse operatives go on strike, and within a week their absence is clearly noticed. They have a direct impact on our lifestyle yet they fall into the lowest order of occupational classification. Conversely, from the highest levels of our social strata, eliminate the lawyer or solicitor, and it is unlikely that their removal from the social scene would have the immediate and universal impact felt by the absence of refuse operatives. The social worth of an occupation is not always attributable to the status ascribed to it. The balance of power is maintained, largely by ensuring that differences in income and wealth continue, irrespective of the extent to which low paid personnel contribute their labour to the prosperity and comfort of society.

To conclude this section we will consider two final issues in relation to social class: the distribution of income and wealth, and the possibilities for moving between social classes; that is, **social mobility**.

The Distribution of Income and Wealth

A refrain from the 1960s 'Money can't buy you love' continues to be heard today as though it contains significance. The success of the national lottery would seem to undermine this sentiment, as millions of people purchase tickets in the hope that they will become multimillionaires, chasing the dream of a secure future and a fantasy lifestyle. The social classes are reinforced by further differentiation in the ownership of wealth. The notions of upper, middle and lower divisions in society become clear when the distribution of income and wealth is considered. The first essential here is to clarify the meaning of the terms income and wealth.

- Income is that money which is gained through work, the State (benefits), and investments.
- Wealth is often referred to as 'marketable assets' . The important issue here is that these goods are kept for their value rather than being essential. For example, owning your own home is not wealth, but owning a second home would be. It is most usual to see wealth expressed in terms of stocks and shares, and land; however, there are many possible variations.

Earlier it was suggested that the divisions between the social classes were blurring, but when the top and bottom income earnings are considered, it is apparent that vast divisions remain. The most wealthy 10% of the population own almost 50% of the total marketable wealth in the country. The most wealthy 50% of the country control 92% of the total marketable wealth. This indicates that the 'other half' of the country owns the remaining 8% of the total marketable wealth. These figures create a graphic image of the divisions evident in the distribution of wealth (Source of figures: Central Statistical Office 1996).

Let us take these issues further and question how such extremes of difference in access to and ownership of wealth and income are maintained. Essentially those at the top of the wealth ladder have existed in that exalted state for many generations, since a large proportion of wealth is inherited. This group is often referred to as an elite group and although small in physical number they exert both political and social power which assists in the maintenance of their position. They represent the majority interest in society, holding the balance of power despite their limited numerical strength. The influence of status and prestige combine with tradition to ensure acceptance by other sections of society so ensuring the maintenance of the status quo.

Within the workplace the hierarchy of authority reinforces social status and imposes a quiet compliance. Reflect back to the discussion on education and it becomes possible to combine the influences of the educational system with those of the workplace. The socialisation processes establish both acceptance of the immediate situation and encourage hope for the future through obedience and hard work. There exist examples of people who have moved upwards in the social sphere through skill, industry and a little bit of luck. Such examples provide an incentive to maintain the social order rather than to challenge it.

Social Mobility

The possibility of improvement is a seductive promise which each individual can strive towards by succeeding in their chosen area of work. The idea of a career is based on an individual's education and work life being directed towards a particular goal which is achieved in stages as time, qualifications and opportunities allow. The career question starts incredibly early in life. We ask children 'what do you want to be when you grow up?' and expect a concrete answer. Utley (1997) reports on research findings from the University of Southampton, by Nick Foskett, that identify that children are making career decisions as early as age ten. The essence of striving is built in as part of early socialisation and is reinforced by career structures in the workplace. The extent to which true mobility exists requires some examination.

The Oxford Mobility study carried out by Goldethorpe and Payne in 1986, surveyed 10 000 men and found that there was indeed movement between the social classes, but this was short-range movement. That is, people find it relatively easy to move up (or down) one or two occupational groupings, but it is very difficult to move, for example, from Goldthorpe's Social Class 7 to Social Class 1. In turn, those who are in Social Class 1 find it relatively easy to remain there. The influence of families and in particular the father provides an imbalanced start in the occupational arena. Fathers in Social Class 1 tend to act as gatekeepers to positions in this highly valued sector; hence the origin of the phrases, 'keeping it in the family' and 'the old boy network'.

Now that we have examined some of the key issues pertinent to the study of the social institutions, some discussion of the relevance of such issues to nursing work follows.

Nursing Work and the Social Institutions

As was outlined in the introduction to this book, nursing is a social activity for which an understanding of the context of care heightens the skills and competence of the nurse. As we begin to see through this chapter, the social world is complex. The internalisation of complex social ideals is promoted through primary and secondary socialisation. Ideas and realities such as family, education and class become regarded as usual, or normative occurrences. When we enter nursing we bring with us our own familiar experiences and feel that we know these complex areas since they have formed part of our lives. Yet nurses have experienced the processes of socialisation, and bring with them taken-for-granted understandings of the social world that require clarification and reflection.

Personal experience of life is insufficient to help the student nurse understand the range of experiences and roles that are likely to become evident over even a short period of time in the practice of nursing. The norms of a society place value on certain aspects of behaviour; such values frequently indicate approval or disapproval. The nurse considers the needs of a wide range of individuals who interpret the world from varying perspectives. It is essential that inadvertent value judgements based on personal socialisation do not impinge on nursing decisions. Additionally, as will be seen in later chapters, individual life experiences have a direct impact on health experiences and potential access to health care.

Changing patterns of family structure are not always found to be good or useful for the functioning of society. Traditional views of the family remain centred on patriarchal values which emphasise the female mothering role and the male provider role. The current changes and variety of family structures are often criticised for placing children at risk through the absence of the mother if she works outside the home or the absence of the father if separated from the family. As Dalley (1988) suggests the role model of the nuclear family remains the measure by which each family is assessed. A secure family, a safe family, a healthy family are defined within parameters which measure closeness to the ideal type, irrespective of the statistical evidence indicating changes in the British family.

The emphasis on the female nurturing role creates particular expectations of the nature of female work and responsibility within the household. Nurses are likely to internalise views such as these to a greater or lesser extent.

The relationship between nurse and client can be positive or negative depending on the interpretation given to the definition of the family. Take as an example a seemingly simple occurrence such as 'visiting time'. It is quite common to see a rule concerning the number of visitors allowed to each bed on a ward. Although the comfort of the invalid and congestion and safety on the ward are important determinants here, the notional number of visitors encouraged for each bed also reflects the expected pattern of the nuclear family. Fewer or greater numbers of visitors can be a source of discussion and lead to judgments being made about the home circumstances of that individual. Such questioning occurs in all areas and branches of nursing where health care and the family touch.

Discussion questions 2.2	All four branches of nursing are concerned with supporting the family to some extent

	Key functions of the family include:
	  Reproduction and sexual activity
	  Child care: Socialisation
	                      Social control
	                      Education
	                      Health and Welfare

	In what ways can you see the nurse being involved with the family in relation to mental health and learning disability nursing?
	Identify commonalities between the four branches of nursing in the ways in which they each both rely on, and provide support for, the family.

As will become clear in later chapters the present system of health-care provision depends on the family and especially the mother, who provides a high percentage of the informal care which supports the health-care system. In the next chapter we will consider some of the differences at the individual level that can impact on the shape and nature of the family and demand that the nurse relinquishes narrowly held ideas.

In the United Kingdom a high level of literacy ability in the general population is taken for granted. Similarly the ability to understand and act on complex instructions is also expected in the client population. A nurse can experience feelings of annoyance when a client fails to respond to instruction in an effective way. Placing such feelings into some balance through remembering the inequalities inherent in opportunities to experience education will contribute towards the development of a more positive nurse–patient relationship. The nurse must develop skills in patient/client education. Such work should recognise the differences in educational opportunity that may influence attitudes towards any other educational enterprise. Perhaps at this point it is pertinent to recall the study entitled 'Pygmalion in the classroom' and remember that ability can be hidden by official classifications or prejudices.

A useful link between education, the family and social class is to consider for a moment the reaction of a nurse on first meeting a new client. As human beings we make many assumptions about the world, not least of these being our definitions of other people. There are many ways that this is accomplished: dress, manner, possessions and speech are among the most commonly used tools to place someone into a notional category box. These categories can be used to assign the social class of an individual and in so doing predetermine many aspects of interaction, the degree of cooperation expected and, far from least, the extent of understanding of medical conditions (Armstrong 1989, Hart 1985, Naidoo & Wills 1994). An awareness of the educational system does help the nurse overcome such barriers to truly seeing the client as an individual. Literacy levels are of restricted value when used as an indicator of ability; they should act only as a measure of opportunity (Doak et al 1996).

The latter is particularly valid when working with clients who have a learning disability. Nurses usually expect a limited range of literacy within this client group, and because there is some intellectual impairment evident, the potential abilities of the client can remain untapped. The combination of prejudgment, low nursing expectations and a restricted exposure to formal education can lead to the client being excluded from

Discussion questions 2.3

How can an understanding of the sociology of the family, education and social class assist the nurse in taking a client history?

How would your understanding of the nature of family help nurses working with people in continuing care? Consider the four branches of nursing in turn.

The social institutions stem from the general foundations of sociological theory; how can the study of sociology improve the nurse's ability to achieve holistic care?

experiences as diverse as conversation through to participation in decision making. An understanding of the social construction of educational ability through the reward system of a social institution should help to limit the prejudgment evident in many health-care areas.

Summary

This chapter has formed a basis for understanding commonly experienced aspects of the social world. The phrase 'social institution' has been introduced and defined. The familiar areas of the family, education and social class have been examined and considered within the context of care. A range of new words have been introduced which have particular meanings in the field of sociology.

Reflection point 2.4

Consider the concepts meritocracy and credentialism.

How may the emphasis on educational achievement contribute to the negative labelling and stereotyping evident towards people with a learning disability?

Some points to consider include:
The status of 'special schools' in the league tables.
The link between status and prestige of employment and any educational prerequisites.

As Community Care develops into a major part of health and social services the function of the family as care provider is re-established. Consider the significance of changing family structures for the provision of community mental-health services.

Some points to consider include:
An ageing population
Divorce and single parenting
Geographical mobility and reduced practical support from local kin

Further Reading

Dalley G 1988 Ideologies of caring rethinking community and collectivism. Macmillan, Basingstoke

This book is a feminist critique of the family that emphasises the degree to which the culture of individualism evolved through capitalism and created a subordinate role for women. You may find pages 28–36 sufficient for your first read.

Fletcher R 1973 The family and marriage in Britain. Pelican, Harmondsworth

Fletcher provides a good historical review of the family in Britain. Although written in the 1970s it remains a useful background to any reflection on the family. Perhaps the romanticism of the past can be dispelled by his reality-based descriptions of family life balancing some of the communitarian idylls of family.

References

Armstrong D 1989 An outline of sociology as applied to medicine, 3rd edn. Wright, Sevenoaks, Kent

Bayley R (ed) 1997 Impact statements go global in Family Policy Bulletin. Families and Politics Spring 1997 Family Policy Studies Centre

Bernstein BB 1971 Class codes and control. Routledge and Kegan Paul, London

Central Statistical Office 1996 Social Trends 26. HMSO, London

Dalley G 1988 Ideologies of caring rethinking community and collectivism. Macmillan, Basingstoke

Doak CC, Doak GL, Root JH 1996 Teaching patients with low literacy skills. JB Lippincott, Philadelphia

Douglas JWB 1969 The home and the school: a study of ability and attainment in the Primary School. Penguin, Harmondsworth

Finch J, Mason J 1993 Negotiating family responsibilities. Tavistock/Routledge, London

Fletcher R 1973 The family and marriage in Britain. Pelican, Harmondsworth

Glendinning C, Millar J (eds) 1992 Women and poverty in Britain the 1990s. Harvester Wheatsheaf, New York, London

Goldthorpe JH, Hope K 1974 The social grading of occupations: a new approach and scale. Clarendon, Oxford

Goldthorpe JH, Payne C 1986 Trends in intergenerational class mobility in England and Wales 1972–1983. Sociology 20

Hart N 1985 The sociology of health and medicine. Causeway Press, Ormskirk, Lancs

Joshi H 1992 The cost of caring. In: Glendinning C, Millar J (eds) Women and poverty in Britain the 1990s. Harvester Wheatsheaf, New York, London, ch 8

Kelly G 1995 Off-the-self sociology. Times Higher Education Supplement 24 March p.21

Labov W 1973 The logic of non-standard English. In: Keddie N (ed) Tinker, tailor . . . the myth of cultural deprivation. Penguin, Harmondsworth

Laing RD 1965 The divided self. Penguin, Harmondsworth

Maynard M 1985 Contemporary housework and the houseworker role. In: Salaman G (ed) Work, culture and society. Open University Press, Milton Keynes

Naidoo J, Wills J 1994 Health promotion foundations for practice. Baillière Tindall, London, Philadelphia

Ormerod P, Rowthorn R 1997 Why family ties bind the nation. The Times Higher Education Supplement 29 August p 16

Rosenthal R, Jacobson L 1968 Pygmalion in the classroom. Holt Rinehart & Winston, New York

Utley A 1997 Poor respond to campus taster. Times Higher Education Supplement, 29 August: 5

Watts AG 1985 Education and employment: the traditional bonds. In: Dale R (ed) Education, training and employment: towards a new vocationalism. Pergamon Press, New York

Weeks DR 1972 A glossary of sociological concepts D283 The Sociological Perspective Glossary. The Open University Press, Bucks

Wilmott P, Young P 1969 Family and kinship in East London. Penguin, Harmondsworth

Wilmott P, Young P 1975 The asymmetrical family. Penguin, Harmondsworth

3 Society and the Individual: Gender, 'Race' and Age

Mary Birchenall

Key concepts

- The nature/nurture debate and gender, 'race' and age
- Social construction theory and gender, 'race' and age
- Language and 'race'
- Disappearing childhood
- Caring for people and community perspective

We have considered three of the major social institutions evident in our familiar social life. Some additional and significant variations within society are evident. These seem to be more subtle and at first appear to relate to natural attributes of the human individual. Three key examples form the focus of this chapter; these are **gender**, **'race'** or ethnicity and age. Each of these attributes has a major influence on individual life and health chances, reflecting differences that are in the main visible, frequently unquestioned and appear to have some biological foundation. The appearance of a biological basis for these individual differences gives rise to a degree of acceptance that leads social actors to perceive the roles they play as natural. Significantly, gender, 'race' and age reflect key social groups in our society. There are other aspects of social life that could be included here but we have chosen to concentrate on issues that are central to the sociology of health and nursing.

Nature or Nurture?

Before embarking on any discussion concerning each of the three aspects of individual difference selected as significant, one common and relevant thread requires unravelling. It was mentioned above that gender, 'race', and age have some biological foundations that could influence the way in which such aspects of individual difference are defined. For example, two of the first questions asked by parents at the birth of a child are, 'Is it all right?' and 'Is it a boy or a girl?'. No one really needs to ask the child's age and the parents know their own national origins. As the label boy or girl is ascribed, or given, at birth the notion of a child's development being split by the gender definition seems natural.

It becomes easy to maintain this acceptance of absolute truth in relation to individual differences. Indeed there is a sense of security in knowing who and what you are, and being able to place others appropriately. Life would be very complex if each time we met someone we had to work out every detail about them so that we could relax sufficiently to have a conversation. So having clues that orient us to these aspects of an individual is useful and saves much time and energy in our social life.

Activity 3.1	Consider the last time that you awaited a meeting with new friends or acquaintances: your discussions should help you realise the structure of the social order as being accepted as the natural order.
	What preparations did you make for yourself?
	Did these vary if your meeting is with people of the same or different gender?
	Did you have some expectations of how people might look or act?
	What happens when there is an unexpected event, such as someone arrives in a wheelchair?

Each aspect of individual difference has a biological basis which is influenced by social factors, such as the processes of primary and secondary socialisation. There is a tendency for these 'natural' categories to become confused with the social definitions for that category. Hence, you may have heard expressions such as, 'It's only natural that the woman should make the home and look after the children, and the man should work to support the home.' You may remember that the family, as a traditional unit, had a number of core functions that were seen as necessary to the maintenance of society. Hidden within the functions of the family are gender roles, that appear to be based on the physiological contribution made by men and women to the creation of a child. Biological distinctions have been used as a major distinguishing factor in the social roles of men and women. This is also evident in respect to age and 'race' also, and we will explore each in turn later.

Essentially, such roles are socially constructed; but sometimes these roles become confused with 'the natural order' or biological differences.

Of concern to sociologists is the way in which the processes of socialisation appear to be overwhelmed by this seemingly natural order. The justification of particular ways of living and the emergence of power imbalances have been overlooked and the natural laws have been used to justify social inequalities, since differences between people are attributed to the natural order. The creation of the various roles through the social constructionist perspective is central to this chapter. The impact of a socially constructed status that is accepted as natural has far-reaching implications. The significance will emerge further as each of the key areas selected is examined.

Gender

Gender and sex roles are often spoken about as though the terms were interchangeable. In sociology it is usual to use the term gender rather than the term sex. It is of course more complex than creating a simple division between the character role, gender, and the procreative role, sex, but for now it is a useful boundary to draw. One thing is certain: orienting to a person's gender is important in every society. The nature of the social roles may vary but there is a universal concern with the significance of gender. In our own society the creation of a gender role starts at or even before birth. Infant behaviours that are similar are attributed diverse interpretations depending on whether the child is seen as male or female. In such ways it is possible to see the nuances that develop biologically determined characteristics into socially constructed behaviours.

Doing Gender

Assigning the sex of a child starts as soon as the infant is born. All those around the baby, including doctors and midwives begin the process of 'doing gender', beginning with the naming games. Names are important clues in the social process and are given attributes independent of the person. Some names are clearly linked to men or women, girls or boys; additionally, some names are considered to be strong and others gentle or even insipid. Of course, the significance of particular names changes over time and are as much constructs of society as any other aspect of social life. A child's name is considered an important event and much parental agonising is evident in their endeavours to match the child and the name. You need only glance at the relevant shelves in the book-shop to become aware of the number of publications, made up almost entirely of a dictionary of names, to help the new parent in this important decision. A famous study by Will et al (1976) records the results of a social experiment concerned with the significance of gender identification.

Reflection point 3.1

A brief outline of the study by Will et al (1976)

A group of women were observed, as individuals, playing with a six-month-old baby, who was given a female name and dressed in pink. The women commented on the gentle nature of the child, and interacted in ways that were intended to soothe and maintain calm. A second group of women were observed handling the same baby, but this time dressed in blue and called by a male name. This baby was regarded as rugged and handsome, and was played with in a way that would be stimulating, seeking activity rather than passivity from the baby.

Discuss in small groups the significance of this experiment.

Reflect on whether such an experiment would have a different result if carried out today?

How might a nurse who works with children make assumptions about boy and girl behaviour?

From birth, children are handled and addressed differently, based on their gender. Doctors and other health professionals play their part in this process, referring to boy babies as sturdy or handsome, and girls as dainty or sweet. This is particularly significant as babies tend to be of fairly similar weights irrespective of their biological sex. I have emphasised these early moments in life as there is a view that gender is less significant in this society as we move towards the twenty-first century. Equality between the sexes is seen to be emerging. This will be considered as we look at the processes of gender socialisation and the social context within which children and adults come to terms with their gender identities.

Gender Learning

The patriarchal dominance evident in the development of British society indicates that women and men are likely to experience at best different but most commonly unequal opportunities. Until the early 1980s sociologists could claim that there were clear divisions which worked to advantage men and disadvantage women. Sue Sharpe's research, published in the book 'Just Like A Girl' (1976) was one such text which showed that girls were socialised into expecting limited horizons and taking responsibility for family care. Over 20 years have elapsed since this study and many changes in the social order are claimed, particularly in relation to emerging equalities.

Sharpe revisited her study in the 1990s and found that the attitudes of girls had indeed changed in some areas. Perhaps the most significant change was their attitudes towards marriage and work. Girls in the 1970s saw marriage as a positive 'career' choice although they considered that there would be possibilities for working beyond marriage, but this would most likely end after the birth of their first child. Girls in the 1990s were less inclined to focus on marriage, considering it a limited option, although work would continue not only after marriage should they select that option but also after childbirth. So girls attitudes have changed but have their opportunities? Sharpe writes:

> 'Many schools have anti-sexist and anti-racist policies and there is general endorsement of equal opportunities. In 1991, for the first time, more women than men applied for a university place, although evidence has always shown fewer women than men actually go to university. Women have not made many inroads into areas of work hitherto thought of as 'men's work'; and they still earn considerably less than men. Girls' hopes in education and employment may therefore be curtailed.'
> (Sharpe 1994:300)

Gender socialisation is far from singular and is also a significant attribute for boys who learn their gender roles at early ages just like the girls. Work such as that by Phillips (1993) 'The Trouble With Boys' and Lee (1993) 'Talking Tough: the Fight for Masculinity' have paid attention to the socialisation of boys. If gender is to become less significant in the creation of divisions within our society then attention also needs to be paid to the ways in which boys take up their social roles, both formal and informal. To date, as Sharpe points out, it is women who have demanded change and worked towards it:

> 'So far it has been girls and women who have changed their perceptions and attitudes, made demands in their personal and working lives, adapted themselves in many ways, and are left doing far more than their fair share in the belief that this is a better use of their talents.'
> (Sharpe 1994:302)

The unconscious acceptance of inequalities of experience based on gender has created many tensions in British society. The literature has emphasised the female gender as women's fight for equality. In recent years a 'backlash' has emerged as demands for equality of opportunity for men are voiced. Perhaps this is an example of the patriarchy reasserting itself as men strive to restore their perceived lost status. The quiet industry of society as it reclaims the functional roles of the genders may be visible here. Communitarianism seeks a return to family values although some emphasis is placed on the need for both parents and a strengthening of the caring role of the father. There are concerns that such pressing demands to return to family values are a faintly disguised attempt to reclaim the traditional role of women.

Learning gender roles begins at an early stage and is to a large extent a taken-for-granted part of our lives, to the extent that even the way that an infant is nursed varies from boy to girl. There should be little surprise then that people grow up with a sense that boy/girl behaviour is natural and normal, since the differences are a part of an individual's continuity of experience.

Reflection point 3.2

Given that social roles are learned at an early age through the processes of internalisation and socialisation, consider some of the early images evident in the literature given to children. Ask yourself, 'What is the significance for the readers of literature of the various images used to portray the characters in texts?'

In what ways do the following character roles imply any specific characteristics that may be associated with gender norms? Witch: Fairy: Goblin: Prince: Princess: Hero: Heroine: Stepmother/father: Spy: FBI Agent: Football Coach: Gymnast.

Identify characters in novels and television programmes that comply or contrast with implied gender stereotyping. You may find it interesting to consider the nature of characters who play the part of nurses from a range of branches.

Gender Images in the Media

Sharpe has indicated that there are changes evident in the ways that gender roles are expressed. There is a sense that a greater equality is evident and indeed equal opportunities legislation establishes the rights of all to fair and non-discriminatory opportunities. In turn, the ways in which roles are portrayed in the media should then have minimal identifiable gender divisions.

Some changes have emerged in recent times. For example, early school reading books are required to portray more egalitarian roles, with limited stereotyping of boy/girl roles. Set against this, television continues to have masculine roles as dominant and active and feminine roles as passive and of less note. If the commercials are taken into consideration this trend is emphasised: where important information is given, a male presence or voice-over is used; the softer and provocative images emphasise women's roles. Of particular note is the discrepancy in the amount of exposure evident between men and women in television. There are many more male than female roles presented on the small screen. Additionally, where role stereotyping has adjusted character portrayal, women and girls are shown as moving into a man's world, but there are few examples of men taking on feminine roles. Even programmes such as Grange Hill, from children's TV, and Heartbreak High, aimed at the adolescent, have the male heroic lead, with the female roles often playing the part of moral conscience.

Activity 3.2	Examine advertisements in some newspapers and magazines. Identify any patterns to the imagery that you find being used to sell certain products. Are there gender divisions? You may find that age and 'race' also play a significant role in the selling of commodities. If the idea of equality exists today how can such adverts be not only accepted, but also often successful?

The use of gender stereotyping in advertising is particularly illuminating; it is here that the taken-for-granted nature of gender roles is overtly evident. Even in those advertisements where there is an apparent role reversal it is the impact of this role change that carries the significance of the message. Advertisers are concerned to sell their product and through the medium of such accepted norms as those of gender roles can send messages in a very brief time slot. Remember that adverts on television are only seconds in length, and those on the printed page must have immediate eye impact if they are to succeed. The recognition and use of social norms is therefore significant in the business world.

Tradition and Gender Roles

In British society education is taken for granted as being available to all if they have the ability to benefit from it and perhaps the greatest change in gender roles is evident in the acceptance of women's rights to participate in all aspects of education. Contrasting the present with Sophia Jex-Blake's struggle to be taught in a university in 1860 could lead to a sense of complacency, as today women and men are considered as having equal rights to education. Helena Kennedy (1995) considers just this issue, and finds that although the opportunities seem more egalitarian, the value base given to 'female' style pursuits remains lower. She quotes Professor Jardine who says:

> '... it is a secret fear of many women that if they choose to work on a woman author, or if they take a woman's studies option or answer a feminist question in their examinations they will pay a consequence. On numerous occasions I have been tempted to dissuade a student from choosing a women's topic, because it will earn a lower grade, or will need to be "much better than normal" to gain a good one.'
>
> (Kennedy 1995)

Such differences between male and female roles extend to the work place. Women must work harder, demonstrate higher order skills, and achieve higher marks in qualifying examinations than their male counterparts. This is evident in medicine and higher education. There is a view, even today, that men have larger and possibly better brains than women

Reflection point 3.3	Three extracts are presented below which are separated in time by 120 years; identify their similarities and differences; you may have ideas and experiences of your own to add.

'... there is a great difference in the mental constitution of the two sexes, just as there is in their physical conformation. The power and susceptibilities of women are as noble as those of men; but they are thought to be different and, in particular, it is considered that they have not the same power of intense labour as men are endowed with.... I should regret to see our young females subjected to the severe and incessant work... indispensable to any high attainment in learning. A disregard of such inequality would be fatal to any scheme of public instruction.'
(Lord Neave 1873 cited by Helena Kennedy 1995)

'Woman has ovaries, a uterus: these peculiarities imprison her in her subjectivity, circumscribe her within limits of her own nature. It is often said that she thinks with her glands. Man superbly ignores the fact that his anatomy also includes glands, such as testicles, and that they secrete hormones. He thinks of his body as a direct and normal connection with the world, which he believes he apprehends objectively, whereas he regards the body of woman as a hindrance, a prison, weighed down by everything peculiar to it.'
(Simone de Beauvoir 1972 p 15)

'Masculinity and femininity are not inherent properties of individuals, but are inherent and structural properties of our society, which both condition and arise from social action. Through this social interaction children learn the meanings of sex and gender in their particular society at any time. They learn to position themselves correctly as male or female. ... In many areas of their lives girls and boys (like "femininity" and "masculinity") have been seen and treated in a contrasting relation to one another. In education, training and work, girls encounter a system that is still premised on such gender differences, which not only denies opportunities, but also assigns a lower value to much of what is seen as "feminine".'
(Sharpe 1994 pp 86–88)

(McCrum 1994). The contrasting argument, and certainly more convincing one, is that women are subject to a glass ceiling which limits their getting off the starting blocks in professional and academic life.

Gender and the Family

Domestic labour is a phrase used to describe the work of women in the family home. Work is a term reserved for paid employment, and is rarely used to refer to housework, although this is now recognised as demanding and essential for the national economy. As Sharpe reported, girls expect to enter the world of work, but they anticipate combining paid employment with the responsibilities of caring for a family. Although there is much said concerning the development of a more equal sharing of work in the home, studies that have investigated this find that there is an absence in the equitable nature of this sharing. Women continue to bear the greater part of the burden of caring for children; this remains true irrespective of the hours worked or the nature of her employment (Berk 1985, Lorber & Farell 1991, Oakley 1985). The role of women in maintaining the family is seen by some as crucial to the maintenance of society, and the absence of the mother from the home is considered a disruption to that social order. So the apparent emancipation of women from the home has been countered by accusations of a dereliction of duty. The continuing role of the mother in child rearing assists in the maintenance of that role as children internalise their observations of gender splits within the family as part of their early socialisation. Of course, the nurturing role is important but this claim is diminished by the absence of an ascribed and socially significant role through status and financial reward.

Women continue to provide a high percentage of the caring services, either formally, paid, or informally, unpaid. In relation to the developments in the provision of community care Dalley (1988) writes:

> 'With women being prepared to remain or return to the home to care, society is provided with a ready-made "reserve army" of nurses... (which) does not need wages to be paid it, because *it is assumed*, its members are already provided for by being dependent on, and thus supported by, wage-earning men.'
> (Dalley 1988:18)

Sharpe recognised in her 1994 study that even though these young girls were focused on a career, those careers remained biased towards the service and caring industries, so maintaining the existing gender divisions within society. These jobs have lower status and this compounds the social status of women. The caring professions do have a noble status in that they are deemed essential and there is some feeling that a special kind of person is needed. In contrast, the level of social significance for such occupations can be measured by the salaries paid to these workers. There remain tensions with the vocational and work-based nature of nursing and its economic value to the State and the individual. Additionally, there are gender divisions within nursing itself where gender roles appear overlaid on professional roles. The significance of gender is evident even in the choices of courses made at University. According to figures reported in the Times Higher Education Supplement (29 August 1997 p 6) three times more women than men study psychology. The reason offered for this difference is that psychology is linked to the caring professions and so attracts a high percentage of women. This is an issue that we will return to later in this chapter.

Gender and Education

As in other areas of social life girls experience education differently from boys (Spender 1982). They are expected to behave in a more feminine fashion and be interested in feminine pursuits such as home economics and the arts rather than science and maths. Some of theses attitudes can be traced to the formative years when the toys selected by parents for their children show some gender divisions (Zammuner 1987). It is suggested that toys for boys are more technical and scientific and have components that require strategic thinking; this makes these areas of the school curriculum familiar to boys who are more likely to succeed in these areas. This reinforces the idea that boys are better at sciences than girls, whose early years of playing have reinforced the girls' future role as mothers or carers. If such early opportunities can create differential skills in children then the notion of the naturalness of gender roles in society can seem even more persuasive.

Spender (1982) proposes another dimension that adds to the impact of gender roles on individual potential development. She highlights that teachers unwittingly give more attention to boys than girls, since if boys do not get what they want they are likely to cause trouble. Frequently, classroom discussions are dominated by boys, and boys are regarded as more worthwhile students than girls. Any endeavours to adjust this imbalance can leave teachers with the feeling that they are being unfair to the boys. This was made evident recently, when data indicated that girls were doing better in GCSE examinations than boys. Figures for the years 1993/94 (Central Statistical Office 1996) show that girls achieved better results in 'A' levels and GCSEs than boys. The immediate reaction was to redress what was seen as an imbalance and do something to help boys in the classroom. This was despite the knowledge that girls have been disadvantaged throughout our history and have greater difficulties in accessing higher education courses than boys.

The above discussions have highlighted some of the principal issues of concern in relation to gender. Frequently the literature has emphasised the female issues. This corresponds to the experience of inequality that is part of the usual lifestyle of women and girls. If your life is at the least balanced and at the best provides you with favourable opportunities you are less likely to research your advantages. Whereas women have for several centuries been fighting towards establishing equality of opportunity and have been concerned to publicise their arguments and research. In the following sections it becomes apparent that the disadvantages built into the structure of our society have wider ramifications. The example of the women's movement has given some encouragement to other groups who have a similar history of disadvantage based on mistaken perception of their ability and the 'natural order of things'. We now move on to consider the extent to which the concept of 'race' is real and develop further understanding of the impact of socialisation processes in relation to the status of particular groups.

'Race'

Recognition of the inequalities of experience and opportunity that permeate British culture demands that each aspect of inequality be confronted. For some nurses their area of work may involve a high percentage of patients from minority ethnic groups, while for others there are few such patients. Both groups of nurses must be aware of the underlying **discrimination** evident in British systems and be able to examine their own internalised values. The start of this process is in understanding the social context of attitudes towards minority ethnic groups and some critical reflection on the concept of 'race'.

The issue of 'race' can create many problems, not least being the use of language. As public sensitivity to the derogatory nature of much of the language used in reference to 'race' has grown, so the political correctness of speech has emerged. At times this arena can seem to be a closely laid minefield that can lead to the temptation to avoid and ignore at all costs. Such a luxury is not permissible in providing healthcare, and some understanding of the impact of social values in relation to 'race' on individual lifestyle and health experience is essential.

Once again the ideas based on biology and naturalness impinge on our understandings. The apparent obviousness of differences, based on skin pigmentation, facial shapes, hair design and language, can lead to denial that the construct of 'race' is an aspect of any given society rather than an attribute of the natural order.

The terms used about people are often indicators of the value placed on that person. Although at times some tenderness can be found in seemingly derogatory words spoken in a gentle tone, it is more usual for the nouns or adjectives used to portray some positive or negative image. Such reticence about language can encourage avoidance, but this is not an area where healthworkers and particularly nurses can fruitfully opt out.

Bhiku Parekh writes:

> 'It is pertinent to begin by asking if race is even a useful concept. Essentially it is a biological term and rests on the assumption that mankind can be divided into different groups on the basis of specific biological properties.... [A]s a result of racial intermingling over the centuries, no pure races can be found. Further, biological properties such as colour of skin, texture of hair and shape of nose or cheek bones obviously do not *cause* the behaviour of the people these properties belong to.'
> (Parekh 1982:5)

This quote not only challenges the use of the term 'race' but also questions the meaning of the word. Again the issue of biological origins is evident in the potential for prejudgements concerning the nature of people based on visible and outward signs. The history of slavery with its abuse of people who were perceived as being 'uncivilised' is uncomfortably ingrained in some of the attitudes and values represented in white culture. Linked to this is the recent modern history of immigration, an occurrence that exacerbated some prejudices concerning minority ethnic groups and their social status. Even in the present day, tensions are evident in cities where 'troubles' are defined through ideas of 'racial tension', and public statements concerning strengthening immigration laws are frequently reported in the media. This section begins by looking at the use of language, moves on to the history of immigration and then to the impact of prejudice on the life chances of minority ethnic groups.

Language

'Sticks and stone may break my bones but words can never harm me' goes an old skipping rhyme. The reality is that words can wound as deep and at times deeper than physical hurt. Words can also create effective barriers that prevent opportunities for communication across those barriers. The most pejorative words are barred by legal statute. This does not ensure that all use of such terms are prohibited; indeed a court case based solely on the use of a single term would seem unlikely. The sensitivity to language that is now current and is often referred to as 'political correctness' can mean that avoidance is the first resort to this subject of 'race'.

The terminology that is common to this area includes the following words:

Race	Discrimination
Racism	Ethnic
Prejudice	Minority
Racial prejudice	Black/Asian

Each term is briefly examined below as clarity in the use of language is essential in this area.

'**Race**' refers to attempts to create homogeneous groups of nations as recognisable sets of people who share looks and behaviours. The external appearance of individuals is not constant across or within nation states, nor can internal features be rationalised to create races. There is as great an internal diversity within groups that share the same outward physical characteristics as exists between groups of dissimilar physical appearance. A brief review of any individual circle of acquaintances will reveal the reality of the diverse nature of any group. Yet the language in popular use continues to claim that specific characteristics are identifiable. Consider, for example, the phrase 'she was a typically Irish colleen' – a statement intended to convey images to the hearer. As the science of genetics develops the reality of a common ancestry has become established. There is only one 'race', the human race. In this book the word 'race' will be used at times but will always be written in inverted commas so recognising the tensions evident in such a notion.

Racism takes the belief that individual races exist a step further, by attributing inferior and superior status to some. The establishing of superiority creates tensions between groups as advantages are given to the 'superior' group to the disadvantage of others. A racist will insist that personality traits or visible behaviours are attributable to some biological foundation. The incidence of a high percentage of white students' success at university is taken as very strong evidence of the accuracy of the superiority thesis. Such beliefs ignore inequalities of opportunity and the apparent 'failure' to succeed by socially accepted measures is taken to justify the label 'inferior'. Interestingly, Social Trends 26 (Central Statistical Office 1996:69) indicates that 'Both men and women from the Black ethnic group are more likely than those of White ethnic origin to have a qualification.'

Prejudice refers to the opinions and attitudes that members of one group hold towards another. Such opinions often have no foundation in truth and are likely to be based on hearsay. Prejudice can lead to favourable opportunities being given to approved groups often to the disadvantage of others. **Racial prejudice** is evident when people are devalued simply on the basis of belonging to a particular ethnic group.

Discrimination refers to the activities and behaviour of people as a consequence of prejudicial values. Discriminatory action occurs when individuals, who for example apply for a job, are measured by their physical appearance or accent rather than their qualifications. This can result in someone who is Indian or Afro-Caribbean being denied a post which is given later to a 'white' person. The inequalities of opportunity in education, outlined in the last chapter, can create a situation whereby discrimination exists at an institutional level – institutional discrimination. Such discrimination may be a factor in the anomaly evident between the high incidence of qualifications (educational or work-related) among the Black ethnic group and their employment prospects: only 57% of the male Black working population were in employment compared to 77% of the male white ethnic group in 1995 (Central Statistical Office 1996).

Ethnic is a term used to denote a specific national group. All human beings have some form of ethnic culture. Standard jokes about British ethnicity often involve a Scotsman, an Englishman and Irishman, the punchline being dependent on prejudices concerning the taken-for-granted attributes of each group. 'Ethnic minorities' refers to those groups of people who share a culture that is markedly different from the dominant group in any particular society. In this text, the phrase 'minority ethnic' group has been selected as the most appropriate phrase to aid this discussion.

Minority groups have a number of characteristics in common; the status of minority has four main constituents.

1. Discrimination is evident in the ways in which they are treated in a given society.
2. Membership of a minority group leads to some sense of solidarity or belonging. This can frequently occur as a consequence of discriminatory acts that lead to strangers supporting each other as a consequence of a mutual recognition of their belonging to a similar minority group.
3. Minority groups are often set apart from mainstream groups in society, through culture and geography. It is not uncommon for minority groups to live in the same part of a city, and to create social and cultural barriers to intermingling with the dominant culture.
4. Minority status refers to the imbalance of power that exists in any society.

In sociological terms the word minority does not necessarily refer to a numerical status. For example, the role of women can be used as a specific example because they have a minority status in British culture, yet they are numerically similar to men. This contradiction, implicit in the use of the term minority, can seem to confuse the issue. In turn, the use of the phrase 'minority status' to clarify the consequences of prejudice and discrimination as being based in the establishment of powerlessness clearly indicates the meaning of minority status for many groups in this society. These issues will be explored more extensively later and especially in the chapters on inequality.

Black/Asian: these two words can create tension in ordinary dialogue and give rise to some tongue-tied reticence on the subject of 'race'. Since the prohibitions on discriminatory language, some words are no longer seen as appropriate. An example of such a word is 'nigger'. The unquoted use of this word would seem shocking in a text such as this, but this is an important indication of changes in language. An example of these changes can be found if video footage of serious BBC programmes such as 'Panorama' are reviewed. In the 1950s this now pejorative word was used in programmes about Black people, not as terms of deliberate insult but by the 'informed' and educated presenters of the programme. When such footage is seen in the context of the present day, the language jars on the ear and becomes an embarrassment. Language is a powerful determinant of the value attributed to any issue. The unintentional insult that may be offered by careless language is far from acceptable. The acceptance by a society of derogatory terms that are classed as having no intended insult, although the people described by such terms reject them, is a measure of that society's racial awareness.

The terms Black and Asian can at times be used as though they are interchangeable. A brief examination of a global map (Fig. 3.1) will demonstrate the mistaken assumptions evident in such a confusion of terms. As can be seen, people from almost the opposite sides of the world make up those who are referred to as minority ethnic groups. By using the phrase 'minority group' there is a tendency to merge groups of people into one, ignoring the many intragroup differences. In such ways the majority group denies the individuality of minority groups and effectively challenges their identity.

Reflection point 3.4

There are many groups of people who have become part of the immigrant population of the UK. Some groups have fled from persecution, others have been enticed with the promise of a richer lifestyle. Each group has experienced difficulties on arrival in this country. Now their grandchildren and great grandchildren continue to experience difficulties.

Consider some of the reasons that contribute to these difficulties.

Consider the problem from the perspective of the newly arrived immigrant, the third generation individual from an minority ethnic group, and the 'local' White Anglo-Saxon individual.

The National Health Service (NHS) was one of the major services that benefited from the labour of the early immigrants to the UK. The jobs that were offered were low paid and of low status. Such positions reinforced the prejudice that minority ethnic groups and in particular Black people were of a lower social class and had less ability than white people.

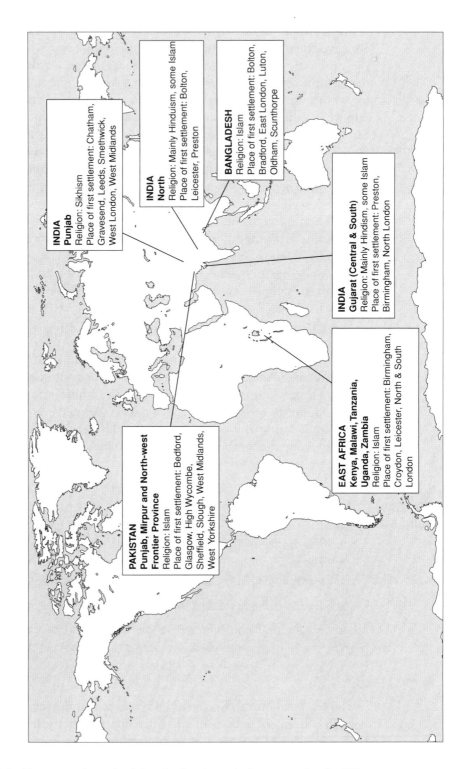

Figure 3.1   The countries of origin of minority ethnic groups in the UK

Today such divisions continue to define the attitudes of the dominant culture, white people, and consequently, have significance for the attainment of responsible positions within the health service.

As with gender, inequalities of opportunity are evident in the experiences of the life for people from minority ethnic groups extending to the workplace. Such inequalities are often masked by confusion between ability and opportunity. As was seen in Chapter 2 education is regarded as responding to ability: the meritocracy approach. In turn, the prejudice evident at all levels of the system limits the easy passage for minority groups to demonstrate their ability and succeed.

Such apparent 'failure' can seem to justify the uneven representation of people from minority ethnic groups throughout the various employment opportunities. This lack of equality is particularly significant within the NHS. Statistical information can appear to indicate that employment opportunities are good within the NHS, particularly in areas that have a higher than average density of minority ethnic group population. Such data must take account not only of the incidence of employment but also of the status of that employment if a realistic picture of the experiences of minority populations are to be gained.

Despite the actual rate of unemployment and redundancy showing a downward trend, individuals remain fearful of being made redundant. It is, therefore, essential that a reassessment of the prejudices inherent in the British system occurs. It becomes easier to justify discrimination in a structure that appears to be threatening to all. The data used to identify the groups who experience such discrimination must clearly indicate any disparities evident in the ethnicity of those who experience unemployment, redundancy and low paid employment. When a problem seems to be experienced by all groups of the population, the continuation of established prejudicial practices can occur unchallenged. Although the possibility of unemployment is shared by all, the risks are higher for people from minority ethnic groups (Skellington & Morris 1992). Certain groups experience a higher incidence of job insecurity and greater difficulties in achieving employment with good pay. This denies these groups the possibility of establishing key individuals into powerful situations that can lead to the development of advocates within the system.

As will be seen in the section on inequalities in health, when life chances are limited there is a corresponding diminishment in the health chances of impoverished groups. In particular Afro-Caribbean people, for whom the differences from the dominant groups are emphasised, experience both personal and institutional discrimination. As Gordon writes:

'It is Black people who suffer the degradation, the injustices and the threats to their security of the immigration control system. They who are

required to produce their passports to establish their immigration status and the legality of their presence here when they claim benefits or seek services. They who are attacked in their homes, schools and public places because of their physical appearance. They who are regarded by people in authority, and portrayed in the press, as an alien threat from which the rest of society must be defended. This is the reality of racism in Britain in the late 1980s, a reality which contradicts any rhetoric of equality or equal opportunities.'
   (Gordon 1989:26)

This expression of racism and prejudice occurs despite the legislation that exists to outlaw such practices. The requirement that organisations present their actions within an equality of opportunity principle remains rhetoric, that is well spoken intentions rather than hard action (Troyna & Hatcher 1992). Equal opportunity policies are too often checklists that fail to challenge in-built prejudice and discrimination. A critical example of prejudice in the educational system was identified by Tomlinson (1983) in her study of 'Special' schools. She found that, in the early 1980s, Afro-Caribbean people were five times more likely than other groups to be placed in 'special' education. She also found that gender was significant, with a higher incidence of boys being sent to 'Special' school than girls. She linked this to the increased likelihood of Black males being located in disruptive units. Interestingly, Asian pupils whose IQ scores were relatively low remained in mainstream education. Tomlinson attributed this to the fear of personal harm when Black students did not conform to the passive student role. Black students were considered disruptive, whereas the Asian pupil, who exhibited the white culture's required passivity, was regarded as unproblematic to mainstream education. The Swann report (DES 1985) 'Education For All' was a significant milestone in uncovering the extent to which racism affects the education of minority ethnic groups. Today the traditions of 'white supremacy' continue to impede the evolution of an equal society. The visible differences of skin pigmentation cloud the common humanity of social actors, reinforcing inequalities.

Later chapters consider the impact of such inequality on individual health status and the experience of health services. Living in an apparently open society such as Britain it can be difficult to comprehend the extent to which individual differences can predetermine individual potential and so opportunity. Denial of racist attitudes is not unusual, particularly in geographical localities that are predominantly white. Graffiti daubed around many locations provide evidence of strong racist feelings frequently among young people. Audrey Thompson (1997) reports the findings of a National Youth Agency project that challenges the overtly racist attitudes of young people in Bermondsey, London.

Reflection point 3.5

Audrey Thompson (1997:19) writes:

'The three year project, funded by the National Youth Agency, worked in an area where racist attacks are so routine that Black and ethnic minority people dare not leave their homes at night. It began at a time when the murders of Stephen Lawrence, the Black teenager stabbed while waiting at a bus stop, Rolan Adams and Rohit Duggal were still very fresh in the popular mind. . . .

At the end of the project, the police were reporting a drop of almost 50 per cent in racist crime in the area. . . .

Kamara (a project worker) says: "The majority of the young people, I would say, did not change. All the work we did on the project would be immediately undone when these people went home."'

How can such life experiences affect the health of people? Points to consider include: Access to health services if the streets are unsafe; stress of living in fear. Consider also the impact of such a violent environment on health-care staff.

Racist attitudes extended from graffiti, 'Vote BNP' posters on walls and fences, etc., to actual physical abuse – stoning and violent attacks leading to hospitalisation.

It is essential for nurses, and others working with people often at their most vulnerable, to reflect carefully on personal decisions, and to identify the hidden assumptions in relation to individual differences that may be present. The health services have attempted to combat racism through a number of reports outlining minimum standards. Not withstanding such documents, the experience of Black nurses remains problematic, as is powerfully reflected in Yasmin Alibhai's (1993) account of three generations of Black nurses. This short biography airs the hopes and aspirations of May, who came in 1949 as an immigrant to Britain to train as a nurse; this is a career also chosen by her daughter and grandaughter, who found the extremes of racism so overwhelming that they advise their children against a career in nursing. Alibhai concludes:

'On the whole, the approach in the health service is overwhelmingly colour blind, and managers reject allegations of racism by claiming all the evidence is anecdotal, exaggerated and impressionistic. They can make this claim, because the DHS has not so far instituted a central ethnic monitoring system which would give a clear national picture. A number of recent reports, however, looking at specific areas show clear trends, and that race discrimination is prevalent throughout the service.'
(Alibhai 1993:105–106)

Age

It is possible that the reader may accept that gender and 'race' are constructed by society. For some this acceptance may be reluctant and for others it is based on personal or friends' experiences. These two aspects of humanity, gender and 'race' are large and feature widely in the media as potential 'social problems'. The area of difference that must be considered next – age – is perhaps more difficult to comprehend as a socially constructed phenomenon.

If any aspect of society appears 'natural' then this distinction would seem to belong to that of age, and perhaps the two extremes of childhood and old age in particular. Surely the various stages of life expressed through the status of infant, child, adult and perhaps elderly or aged person can be regarded as a natural aspect of life? All humans share the experience of being newly born, but the significance of that status varies between societies and over time. We will briefly consider this aspect of social reality and then move on to reflect on the impact of membership of a social group to the work of those in health care.

A Brief History of Childhood

Childhood is a particular aspect of human experience; an historical review can illuminate the nature of the social construction of this phenomenon. The historical work of Aries (1973) effectively illustrates the changes in the role of the child over centuries. He documents the emergence of childhood as a relatively modern concept.

Let us examine further the idea of childhood as a new phenomenon. Before the nineteenth century the survival of infants and young children was uncertain and the social response to this was to create an extended infancy. For approximately the first five years of life, children – both boys and girls – were treated as sexless infants and dressed in similar gowns. It was quite common for the naming of the child to be delayed until survival could be expected. On being named the child portrayed the role of little man or little woman. Family portraits and diaries of these earlier centuries provide insights into the ways in which the developmental years were very different prior to the twentieth century. In these paintings the solemnity of the young person, parodying the sobriety of the adult is evident. In the society of the Royal Courts it was common to employ adult 'dwarves' as companions for children, reinforcing the notion of the 'little man or woman'. So for most of our history, childhood as we know it did not exist.

Even in relatively recent times, young children were sent out to work often undertaking dangerous life-threatening jobs, in mines, factories and other places of employment. Details of some of the working conditions of children are evident in famous Victorian literature, in stories about such activities as street sellers (The Little Matchstick Girl) or chimney sweeps (The Water Babies). The nurturing component of caring for children is not owned specifically by society in the present, parental love existed at all times in history. On the other hand, when the survival of the family unit is dependent on the work of the entire family then the luxury of childhood was an understandable if unattractive absence. The special status of the child is a creation of modern times.

In the twentieth century the emphasis has been on the vulnerability of the child. Developments in education, particularly during the last 50 years have extended childhood. In earlier centuries, education was reserved for the adult (Aries 1973). Presently, the emergent role of the child has required that longer time periods are spent in dependent mode in educational institutions. As employment laws and opportunities change, then school years became longer for all social classes.

Two conflicting developments are evident in the present day: these are characterised by the extension of childhood through education and the earlier achievement of adulthood when the age of majority was reduced to 18 years. The achievement of education for all was seen as a major social advance. The links between education and future prospects made education a positive experience. Up to the late 1970s the school leaver could look forward to a range of opportunities in the workplace. From the 1980s to the present day this has changed and the role of education has further evolved.

The use of the school to maintain the dependence of young people has been created as a consequence of the reductions in present employment possibilities. The expectations of young people to aspire to independence and take up the trappings of adulthood are evident in the many frustrations visited on the social system by teenagers, and some not yet into their teens. This limbo in the experience of achieving adulthood in our society is one that is specific to this time.

The transition from child to adult is marked in any society by some

Reflection point 3.6

Fact File taken from The Times Higher Education Supplement (August 1997:2)

'The Higher Education Statistics Agency findings for 1995/96 reveal that:

- Unemployment is the first destination of 5 per cent of those qualifying at postgraduate level
- Unemployment is the first destination of 10 per cent of those qualifying in combined study postgraduate programmes
- Unemployment is the first destination of 1 per cent of those qualifying in medicine and dentistry.'

form of ritual process, a rite of passage. The reductions in employment opportunities for young people and the extension of education without necessarily improved employment prospects have created real frustrations for the aspiring adult. Additionally, the world of the adult is seen as important and to be gained at any cost, leading to some reductions in the extent of childhood. Statutes may define the legal parameters of the child but it is the socially determined norms that influence the actions of the human individual.

The Erosion of Childhood

The idyllic life of the child is encapsulated in stories written by authors in the 1950s such as Enid Blyton's 'The Famous Five'. Currently, we nurture the idea of childhood innocence and the necessity of protecting and caring for the child. Yet there exist fears that once again the dark ages of childhood are emerging. The almost sacred status of the child has indeed had a very short course in history and there is evidence that childhood is under threat, if not of extinction then at least of abbreviation.

The disappearance of childhood is catalogued very effectively by Postman (1985). He suggests that television has replaced parents and teachers as the gatekeeper for information into the adult world. He considers the expansion in the number of children convicted of adult-style serious crimes as further evidence of the devolution of childhood. Although Postman's research was carried out in America a range of 'famous' crimes have been publicised in this country, perhaps the best known being that of the murder of young Jamie Bulger by two children. There is evidence of increasing car thefts and destruction, and that the elderly population can be held to ransom by gangs of youths.

Activity 3.3

Read the following extract from the verbal warning in relation to the appropriate audience for video programmes, and discuss the significance of the content for the image of the special status of the child. Speculate on the contribution of the 'permissive' society to the possible erosion of childhood.

'This film is unsuitable for anyone younger than 15 ... fairly adult theme or may contain scenes of violence sex or drugs which are unsuitable for younger teenagers. It may also contain some sexual swear words, some sex or violence.'

The question such stories raise is whether TV is the cause of these changes in childhood. There are other significant factors here that must enter into the equation of the disappearing child. Identified above are some 'sins' of children; increasingly, there is evidence that children are also sinned against. There is a growing awareness that children are abused within their families and that the fashions of society create situations that reduce our awareness of child abuse. During 1995/96 there was an emphasis in the fashion world for the 'waif' look; this fashion also presented catwalk and photograph models as pubescent girls with bruised eyes and haunted looks. Such imagery when placed side by side with pictures of war-haunted children from the third world must raise some speculation as to the place of childhood in the present day. Over the last decade, mother-and-daughter, and father-and-son look-alike clothing ranges have prospered. It would seem that the confusion of adult and child is recurring in the present as was noticeable in our earlier history.

The use of drugs and alcohol by ever younger children is a current major concern. Hospital and community services find that their caseloads now include a significant number of children experiencing the negative effects of their addictions. The continued development and advertisement of alchopops requires us to question the status of childhood in modern-day society. The special regard for the child in modern-day society must now be held in question if the determination to exploit them as consumers to the detriment of their health continues.

In turn, the exploitation of the child has other dimensions. Sexual abuse of children is now recognised as being of wider prevalence than our societal image of the child as asexual and nurtured leads us to expect. Extensive use of children in pornographic literature, holidays abroad arranged around the needs of the paedophile, or children as prostitutes in this country are further examples of the changing nature of childhood. A teacher of the author's acquaintance in a comprehensive school, herself in her early twenties, finds the stories of drinking, clubbing and sexual activities, told by a range of school children aged 11–16 years, bewildering. The increasing incidence of childbearing in school-age children indicates some evidence of the growing realities of the erosion of childhood.

Reflection point 3.7

In 1993 3500 teenagers under the age of 16 had live births and a further 3800 had a pregnancy terminated. Of this group 400 were under 13 years of age.

Reflect on the significance of such statistics for the thesis that childhood is disappearing.

Consider the needs of a pregnant adolescent and the potential service dilemmas as to the best place for care and the most appropriate practitioner – children's nurse or midwife?

Source: Central Statistical Office 1996

The Ageing Process

The onset of old age as with childhood has some biological links. The social interpretation of these changes varies considerably. Tracing the onset of old age through two people living at opposite ends of the twentieth century is illuminating. Both young men in the case studies stem from similar lower middle class homes.

The case studies show only two small glimpses of the ways in which the social structure can influence an individual's experience of ageing. The biological processes of ageing are influenced by social considerations. The concept 'old' is not in itself biological, rather it carries with it certain social constructs. These constructs influence the interpretation of 'age' irrespective of individual experiences and variables in personal biology. For example, there are many phrases used that provide short cuts to communication. One such phrase – 'She is very fit and active, for her age' – incorporates the tacit information that fitness and activity are age dependent. The phrase is most often used in relation to someone who is older, that is at a stage of life when physical deterioration is anticipated. It is only in relatively recent times that assumptions about mental frailty being correlated with increasing age have been challenged.

Essentially, individual differences have biological foundations upon which have been built socially constructed roles. Age is characterised through key social roles that have identifiable correspondence to specific stages of life. Gender and 'race' also have socially prescribed roles that appear linked to biology. These roles are found to be variable throughout history and geography. Biological aspects of the human individual may influence some components of the roles but they do not in themselves determine the social interpretation of that role. What is significant is the way in which a society defines certain attributes. There are other differences between individuals that could be considered. For example, you may like to reflect on the way in which ability and disability are defined. The absence of mobility may appear to be clearly linked to physiological determinants, but some thought can highlight ways in which the society influences the experience and interpretation of disability. A society that is dominated by mobile people creates easy access to and through buildings for the upright stance. Finkelstein challenges us to consider a society where the wheelchair bound are dominant and to consider then the shape of, for example, doors. The mobile would find their mobility impaired if door frames were wide and low rather than high and narrow as now. So perhaps you can begin to see how many attributes of the human person can be overlaid by social interpretations rather than exist as significant determinants in their own right.

Case Study 3.1

Joe. Born 1911	Fred. Born 1980
Starts school Autumn 1916	Starts nursery 1983; enters school 'proper' 1984
Completes schooling Summer 1928	Completes secondary education 1998
Enters into an apprenticeship 1928 which he completes in 1933	Gains a place in Further Education 1998 leaving in 2000 with a Btec ONC
Gains employment with the firm he apprenticed to and remains with them until retirement in 1976	Experiences a range of work placements on short-term contracts until 2006 when he gains a post
Retires and takes up an interest in gardening and fishing	Made redundant in 2016. Remains unemployed, participating in retraining programmes, etc. until 2020
1981 Has a cerebral vascular accident (stroke) and is left with some paralysis	2020 Gains a number of different jobs until 2036
1983 Attends a day centre to receive day-care and becomes an old man	Remains a 'job-seeker' but registers on a number of educational opportunities entitled 'Training for a Healthy Retirement'
Experiences life as a lonely and inactive old man who is thought to have nothing to contribute to society	2040 Officially reaches retirement age and enters a new stage of life. Becomes active in a society dedicated to 'elder empowerment'
Dies alone, 1996. His body is not found for several days, until the ambulance driver decides to check on his non-attendance at the centre	Enjoys retirement, remains fit and active until late 80s when his vision becomes impaired. Dies 2081

Review the two case histories above, and consider the significance of the differential experiences of employment of these two men. If you work in groups you can add details to these cases, such as marriage/divorce and create different scenarios by varying the social class and economic situation of the two people.

Caring for People

The need for nursing and other care staff to consider the individual is paramount. Ideas about individualised care are accepted as the normal practice. Yet society as a whole has some difficulties in regarding the individual, having many taken-for-granted assumptions about the abilities of people linked to predetermined ideas. As members of this society many of these assumptions form part of our internalised wisdom and it requires deliberate reflection and personal evaluation to examine our own prejudices. These prejudices may even feel 'right' rather than appearing as pre-judgements.

An understanding of the ways in which society has been constructed will help in the development of individualised care and avoid the trap of making assumptions about people based on preconceived ideas linked to the status of gender, 'race' or age. Society can appear as an anonymous catch-all for many limitations, but it is important to remember that we are all members of society and contribute to its construction in some way.

Activity 3.4

Imagine a GP reception area: for example, the layout, the facilities provided for patients and the reception desk itself. In what ways does this major provider of health care take account of individual differences?

You could develop a questionnaire based on some of the ideas in this and other chapters to examine some of the many areas needed to achieve an individualised care approach.

Move your thinking through a range of needs including gender, 'race' and age. You might like to extend your thinking to disability.

Of course, the constructs of gender, 'race' and age do not exist in isolation from each other. Each individual experiences social life from the perspective of all three constructs. Some will find no difficulties in life that can be attributed to their gender, 'race' or age others will find greater significance in one or all of these ideas. Thinking back to the previous chapter, in which we examined issues such as equality and social class, you can begin to extrapolate some of the complex links that emerge from apparently simple ideas such as gender. In 1993, writing in the foreword of Miriam Bernard and Kathy Meade's (1993) book, The Right Honourable Barbara Castle states:

'I do not like writing about being old. This is no doubt partly vanity – we all tend to think of ourselves as perennially young, but partly because society too has such a negative image of what it is like to be old.

But it is also that the subject bores me. I am never conscious of being old, merely of not being able to see very well or take my dogs for as long walks as I used to, or to do much gardening. Otherwise my life style remains broadly unchanged. . . .

Of course, I am one of the lucky ones. . . .

I am well aware that women on the whole are among the most disadvantaged of our society. It has been my pride and joy to use my political position to help remedy that. The Equal Pay Act, which I got through Parliament in 1970, was far from perfect but it was a breakthrough, establishing the right of equal pay by law for the first time in our history. . . .'

It is essential that issues such as gender, 'race' and age are seen as part of a life-span approach rather than as brief snapshots in time. The individual who is disadvantaged by his or her gender can have this disadvantage compounded by his or her 'race' and age. Disadvantage rarely occurs in a single area of life and is often reflected in many key aspects of social life including education, employment, social and economic status. For individualised care which takes account of holistic needs the process can now be seen to be more complex than on initial examination.

Community Perspectives

As care services move from the illness-based traditions of the hospital towards a community and health-promotional bias, the significance of population studies is emerging. Community-health initiatives focus on the needs of local groups rather the individual. National populations are targeted through mediums, such as the 1992 Health of the Nation report (DoH 1992). At a global level the World Health Organisation sets worldwide targets for health. Public health emerged as a major feature of health services with the realisation that attention to social and environmental aspects of human experience improved the health of the population beyond the scope of individual medical care. Currently, population health research is an emerging science. At the level of the practitioner it is linked to the emphasis on health education. Consider, for example, the role of the health visitor in maintaining a watching brief on the health of vulnerable members of the population.

Studying the individual in society is complex. The few examples offered within the scope of this book begin to show the multiplicity of experiences that are part of social life. Such experiences cannot be divorced from perceptions about health and the health services. In nursing there is some tension between the nature of individualised care, holistic care and community health education. The concept of 'age' provides a useful medium for examining the nature of this tension. As already noted, age is as much social construction as biological inevitability. The interaction between the biological, social and psychological aspects of individual life within any particular environment contribute to the experience of ageing. As recently as the late 1960s age was considered to be inevitably a period of physical and intellectual deterioration (Riley 1993). This seemed to indicate that senility was a 'natural' component of ageing. Population health research demonstrates that such assumptions are inaccurate and reflect prejudice rather than biological or psychological reality (Riley 1993).

Understandings of disease and health are well defined in the present day. Public health has progressed through alliance with some theories of social science. The renewal of population studies offers the potential for elaborating on the factors that influence health beyond the biological (Dean et al 1993). Such developments in the theory of health have an impact on the practice of nursing as can be seen by the responses to government initiatives aimed at reducing known diseases and negative health states.

Summary

This chapter has reviewed three significant aspects of individual life: gender, 'race' and age. We have reflected on the impact of the social environment and social norms in the creation of these three aspects of human life. Challenges have been stated with regard to the impact of taken-for-granted assumptions concerning the natural basis of inequalities in our society. The significance of individual experiences of socialisation that define the attributes gender, 'race' and age were considered in the final section. Additionally, a brief reflection was offered on the changing nature of health services from an individual focus to community and population emphasis.

Further Reading

Skellington R, Morris P 1992 'Race' in Britain today. Sage Publications, London

This is a useful overview of particular relevance to health-care workers who seek more knowledge in this area. There are chapters giving details of health experiences alongside chapters on social 'problems' linked to the idea of 'race'.

Scraton P (ed) 1997 'Childhood' in 'crisis'? UCL Press, London

This book is of particular relevance to those who work with children. It takes a critical look at the world of the child and reviews some of the current legislation and responses to policy. As an edited text it is particularly useful when you are searching for a different angle on some of the perennial problems in child care.

Oakley A 1985 Sex, gender and society. Revised Edition. Gower, Aldershot
This book remains a useful and relevant general text on the sociology of gender, written from a feminist perspective. Some cross-cultural studies are included alongside reflections on gender particular to Western cultures.

References

Alibhai Y 1993 Black nightingales. In: Walmsley J et al (eds) Health welfare and practice reflecting on roles and relationships. Sage Publications, London, ch 16

Aries P 1973 Centuries of childhood. Penguin, Harmondsworth

Beauvoir de S 1972 The second sex. Penguin, Harmondsworth

Bernard M, Meade K (eds) 1993 Women come of age. Edward Arnold, London

Berk SF 1985 The gender factory: the apportionment of work in American households. Plenum, New York

Central Statistical Office 1996 Social Trends 26. HMSO, London

Coles B 1985 Gonna tear your play house down: towards re-constructing a sociology of youth. The Social Science Teacher 15(3): 78–80

Dalley G 1988 Ideologies of caring: rethinking community and collectivism. Macmillan, Basingstoke

Dean K, Kreiner S, McQueen DV 1993 Researching population health: new directions. In: Dean K (ed) Population health research linking theory and methods. Sage Publications, London

Department of Education and Science (DES) 1985 Education for all: the report of the committee of inquiry into the education of children from ethnic minority groups. CMND 9453 HMSO, London (The Swann Report)

Department of Health (DoS) 1996 Health of the young nation. HMSO, London

Gordon 1989 Hidden injuries of racism. New Statesman and Society 12: 24–26

Kennedy H 1995 Prisoners of gender. Times Higher Education November 3

Lee C 1993 Talking tough: the fight for masculinity. Arrow Books, London

Lorber J, Farrell SA (eds) 1991 The social construction of gender. Sage Publications, Newbury Park

McCrum NG 1994 The academic gender deficit at Oxford and Cambridge. Oxford Review of Education 20(1): 3–26

Oakley A 1985 Sex, gender and society, revised edition. Gower, Aldershot

Parekh B 1982 The experience of Black minorities in Britain. Open University Press

Philips A 1993 The trouble with boys. Pandora, London

Postman N 1985 The disappearance of childhood: how TV is changing children's lives. WH Allen, London

Riley MW 1993 A theoretical basis for research on health. In: Dean K (ed) Population health research linking theory and methods. Sage Publications, London

Sharpe S 1976 Just like a girl. Penguin, Harmondsworth

Sharpe S 1994 Just like a girl. How girls learn to be women from the seventies to the nineties, new edn. Penguin, Harmondsworth

Skellington R, Morris P 1992 'Race' in Britain today. Sage Publications, London

Spender D 1982 Invisible women: the schooling scandal. Writers and Readers, London

Times Higher Educational Supplement 1972 Fact File. August: 2

Tomlinson S 1983 Sociology of special education. Routledge and Kegan Paul, London

Thompson A 1997 Young, gifted and racist. Community Care 1188 (4–10 September): 18–19

Troyna B, Hatcher R 1992 It's only words: understanding 'racial' and racist incidents. New Community 18(3): 493–496

Will J, Self P, Datan N 1976 Maternal behaviour and perceived sex of infant. American Journal of Orthopsychiatry 46

Zammuner VL 1987 Children's sex-role stereotypes: a cross-cultural analysis. In: Shaver P, Hendrick C (eds) Sex and Gender. Sage Publications, London

4 Introducing Theory in Sociology

Mary Birchenall

Sociology is complex but can masquerade as simple. For example, social commentary can seem complicated when describing social interactions at a societal level but appear straightforward in relation to familiar notions such as the family.

The emphasis of this book is to introduce the social context of nursing and health care. The purpose of this chapter is to provide the new student of sociology in the nursing curriculum with some information about the theoretical underpinnings of a major science, so that the relevance of sociology to nursing practice and health care can be understood and appreciated.

Sociology, in common with any other science, has its own use of language which contributes to interpretations of significant events. Frequently, when an area such as health care is studied for the first time, novice practitioners are met with texts which assume some familiarity with the 'mysteries' of **sociological theory** and understandings of the world. So, before engaging with the key factors which may seem to be at the centre of a sociology of health, an introduction to the sociology of everyday life formed the early chapters of this book. A sociology of everyday life incorporates such apparently ordinary features as the family, education, gender and age. Additionally, concepts such as social class and 'race' were found to be important influences on our understanding of individualised care.

What is Sociology?

A common starting point when exploring a new subject is the presentation of a definition. To define sociology and so give it some absolute meaning is an exercise to be undertaken with some caution. One starting point is the statements made by other authors; from there will develop the meaning for this text and a tentative proposal for the meaning of sociology for nursing. Three definitions, taken from popular introductory textbooks, are listed below followed by some consideration of each in relation to nursing and health care.

'Sociology is the systematic study of societies.' (O'Donnell 1992). Haralambos (1980) proposes that humans are singular in the animal world in that they are dependent on the need to 'learn the culture of its society'; having no genetically determined behavioural patterns, all must be learned. He then elaborates on this, identifying the differences which exist in the known social world, using extremes to elaborate the discussion.

Giddens defines sociology as '. . . the study of human and social life, groups and societies . . . The scope of sociology is extremely wide, ranging from the analysis of passing encounters between individuals in the street up to the investigation of global social processes.' (1997:7–8)

This book intends to be systematic in its approach to the study of nursing and health care. Although nursing may not be seen as a society in itself it is a component part of the society in which we live. It is a common and sometimes useful ploy to use extremes to project an understanding of the everyday events and matters. At times, some examples from extreme circumstances will be used to promote an understanding of nursing events and relationships. The sociology of nursing and health care has a wide range of study. Potentially, to gain insights into practice the actions of only one person need be studied; this can be extended up to whole populations' experiences of health and health care. Comparisons can be made between wards in a hospital, electoral wards in communities, cities, counties and, today, even nations. So a sociology of nursing and health care can encompass actions at the level of the individual and at the level of populations. Increasingly, health initiatives and experiences have impact at a global level, so the need to see beyond narrow horizons is important.

A brief consideration of three commonly used definitions of sociology underlines the complex nature of the study of society and the people who populate that society. It is difficult to capture such notions in the proverbial nutshell. Additionally, there is no one truth as to what sociology is about; studies of society and people require that a discourse emerges that reviews the many variables that contribute to the creation of any one event in any one time. Additionally, concepts of time and place must be considered: no event occurs in a social vacuum. One constant emerges:

sociology is about people, the ways in which they live and the 'why' of those choices. The degrees of difference are representative of the ways in which social scientists approach the study of people and society, and develop theoretical perspectives concerning the nature of the social world.

It should now come as no surprise that the ideas presented by sociologists on such everyday phenomena as the 'family' or 'education' can vary to the point of appearing to contradict, depending on their theoretical stance or perspective. Further elaboration of some key sociological perspectives will help to develop an understanding of this complex nature, and create the platform through which to portray a sociology of nursing. In this way a route towards evolving a definition of sociology for yourself can emerge and this, in turn, can avoid prescriptive sentences which cannot capture the breadth of the essence of sociology.

Perspectives in Sociology

For the newcomer to this area of study there could be some confusion when reading the remainder of this text if it overlooked an introduction to the theoretical differences which colour the approaches towards investigating society and subsequently the literature produced.

Discussion point 4.1

In small groups list any theories that are known to your group members. You may then consider their relative significance in your lives and the degree to which they may widely known in society.

Points to consider: theories of ability in relation to gender, age and 'race' exist. We also have ideas of 'old wives' tales' that can be viewed by some as extracts of wisdom.

The study of sociology has evolved in recent times to such a degree that the espousal of separate theories in absolute opposition to each other is seen in an unfavourable light. For the sophisticated reader familiar with the nature of the works of the 'Founding Fathers' and current writings this would be no surprise. Those coming to sociology for the first time may have expected some right or wrong answers.

This necessarily short overview of theory will avoid the approach that provides a quick tour of key authors under related perspectives. First we will examine the nature of a theoretical perspective and then consider two main divisions in approaches to understanding the theoretical presentations of writers and researchers. As some understanding of the perspectives develop links with nursing and health-care research will be made.

'What is Sociological Theory?'

This question is posed by Mary Maynard (1989) who writes in response to her own question:

> 'At its most simple, sociological theory involves exploring the relationships between different areas and kinds of social life. It is concerned with the conditions under which certain processes and patterns of structure or conflict are likely to occur. It involves classifying aspects of the social world, providing an understanding of them and looking for the causes of and explanations for them.'
> (Maynard 1989:4)

The key words in the quote taken form Maynard (1989) are, *relationships, classifications, understanding, causes* and *explanations*. These concepts are important for any theory, including nursing theories. You should check the meaning of these words before you progress further. Each time that a theoretical understanding is referred to, each of these ideas will be implicit.

Traditionally, sociology has been somewhat insular, focusing on the immediate society. A reasonable occurrence for a new science, when understandings of the known society were on a commonsense basis in which individuals tried to offer explanations of their own world. Such commonsense ideas are theoretical in themselves but sociological theory demands a more informed and far-seeking approach. For example, it is difficult for individuals to see and examine many of the social systems which influence their lives. Take, for example, the education system which is a complex affair, and requires a methodical approach to study and explain. When links to other social factors such as class, 'race' and gender are to be made, these can be even more difficult to 'see'. This is particularly evident since our commonsense understandings are based in a social setting which we accept and regard as normal. Subsequently, it could be very difficult to identify the ways in which class 'race' and gender can disadvantage some and advantage others. Additionally, the manner in which socially constructed differences such as gender, age and 'race' can be compounded and create multiple discrimination in individual lives must be accounted for in any theory of society.

A sociological study of these structures could demand that we take on board as a 'truth' the opposite of our commonsense understandings. Take, as an example, mathematical skills: for decades it was assumed that as boys did better at maths, they had a more 'natural' aptitude in this area than girls. Sociological studies have shown this to be untrue: girls are as able as boys, but the social structures created conditions within which boys developed their mathematical acuity. So sociology can demand that we re-define truth and can make us feel very uncomfortable when we find that a negative situation is far from 'natural', but has been constructed by our own actions.

A frequent accusation made by adult students of sociology, particularly women, is that 'I was happy until you made me start questioning my life!' In later sections of this book we will consider ways in which we as nurses can construct myths about patients and groups and establish these myths as fact, oblivious to our own contribution in their creation.

It has been usual to introduce sociology as consisting of a number of apparently disparate perspectives which can seem to be in opposition to each other. For example, **Functionalism**, Conflict Theory, **Symbolic interactionism**, Post-Modernism and **Feminism** are some of the most commonly reviewed theories in sociology. By placing authors under particular perspective umbrellas there is the implication that within each group there is agreement. Even the briefest of readings can dispel this idea. As a way of trying to capture the complexity of sociological theory, the listing of perspectives and attribution of authors to a distinct category is not always useful. Further, over time, and as a consequence of changing interests, theorists can change their stance. As this is a text to introduce the sociology of nursing and health care rather than sociological theory a narrower option than a review of the many perspectives is proposed. Sociological theories are presented here as having two main divisions: Structuralism and Interpretivism. Each of the two divisions will be examined and then links to nursing and health care identified.

Structuralism

The early development of this theory is founded in the nineteenth century when the language of the then developing science of biology was used to develop analogies for the social world. In this way terms such as 'structure' and 'function', became features of the description of and, inevitably, the explanations of the social world.

Structuralism, as the word implies, is concerned with structure. When the structure of an artefact is considered the aspects of interest are the ways in which it was constructed, or created, and additionally through which it is maintained. A process of understanding the way in which structure has evolved is undertaken. In a similar manner, the structures of society are of interest to sociological theorists. The ways in which societies are constructed, held together and ordered are of paramount interest to some. For others, the focus of study is understanding the nature of components of that society – such as an organisation, perhaps a hospital – and the ways in which the structure helps or hinders progress, efficiency and effectiveness.

<table>
<tr><td>Reflection
point 4.1</td><td>Consider the nature of a social structure by listing as many structures in your own society as possible.

Divide your list into structures that have direct influence over your life and those that seem more remote.

To what extent are you aware of structural influences in your daily life?</td></tr>
</table>

Consensus and Conflict

The nature of those structures which identify a society or its parts have one other significant aspect which must be considered here: the nature of the internal relationships within the structure. Such relationships are seen to be either consensual or conflicting in their nature. *Consensus* requires a supportive and commonly held aim that works towards the achievement of common social goals. Ideas here are based on *conflict*, and are characterised by antagonistic relations set within an imbalance of power. The idea of two sets of understanding, one based on consensus and the other on conflict, begins to indicate the ways in which there is no real uniformity within the theories brought together under the heading 'structuralism'. The significant features which identify this strand of theory are firstly, the emphasis on social structures, which may vary in scale from large to small; secondly, the demand for an objective view of the world.

A key writer in relation to the demand for a scientific and objective study of the social world is Merton who took the view that the nature of society be tested by empirical research (Merton 1968). Such empirical studies are carried out using a 'scientific' methodology, based on the traditional physical sciences. These physical sciences are often referred to as 'pure' science. Writers such as Durkheim (1970) established the scientific principles which would create a scientific study of society. It is possible that the term 'positivism' may be linked to this form of study and that 'positivism' forms the method of investigation (methodology) preferred within the structuralist framework. Positivism has been defined as 'the science of society', following Comte's early work, and espouses the requirement that social artefacts should be studied objectively using the principles and procedures of science.

Consensus and Conflict Theories

A split is evident in structuralist perspectives; the issue of consensus and conflict are widely debated. The functionalist arguments seek to identify the ways in which social institutions, such as the family or religion, work towards solidifying social relationships. A collective response to what can seem to be the vagaries of social life is seen as contributing to the structures and functioning of society. In contrast, evidence of dysfunction within society could not be overlooked and the potential of disintegration of society through such areas of conflict are also important areas of study for some. Two main traditions of theory are evident here: the functionalist, sometimes referred to as structural functionalist, and the Marxist schools of thought. The ways in which social theorists orient themselves can help to clarify some of the differences in perception which emerge in various writings. Nursing and health care have structures and functions that may dysfunction; these are of interest to us and require explanation and investigation through empirical means.

Activity 4.1	Map out the details that define the organisation which is your place of employment or education; identify its structure.
	Create a diagram to represent the lines of authority that you see as existing.
	Place your self at some point in that diagram, and consider the following questions.
	How do these lines of power affect you?
	Are you always in agreement with the demands of the organisation, whether in action or in thought?
	How do you manage your own feelings of conflict?

To some extent the relative power positions within a society or organisation must have some impact on each individual. Set against this is the idea of scale; at times each individual must feel so far removed from certain authorities that there is a questioning of the reality of that impact from such remote power structures. Perhaps there is the feeling of being a 'free agent' so long as the notice of particular people is avoided. A brief consideration of these issues will bring the realisation that structural power invested in key figures does have an impact on each individual. The process of 'avoiding notice' is an example of such power.

Many organisations have what is termed a 'Mission Statement' which embodies its aims or goals. The extent to which these goals are shared by the membership will determine the degree of consensus that exists. The study of conflict and consensus within an organisation, small or large, is of interest to theorists within the structural domain. Whether their emphasis is consensus or conflict would possibly indicate whether they originated from functionalist (consensus) or Marxist (conflict) perspectives. Essentially, both parties are concerned with an aspect of the structure of an organisation.

Structuralism, as a theoretical stance, can take as a focus for study as small an organisation as a ward, or as broad as the hospital. An even wider arena is possible when societies are taken into account. There exists at present notions of the 'diminishing world'; the globe appears smaller as communication networks and travel potential become easier and swifter. Telecommunications can establish almost simultaneous interaction across the world. Traditionally, sociology has seemed insular, focusing on the study of the immediate society, sometimes making inferences for other but similar parts of the globe. The study of 'exotic' cultures was the domain of anthropology. In turn, the feeling of the diminishing size of the world, through developments in communication and transport, has stimulated a growing interest in the global nature of society. A need has been identified to describe and understand the structures which link nations, and establish hierarchies and power relations, on a worldwide scale.

The study of society and its structures has evolved from earlier ideas of internal function, whether consensual or conflicting in its nature, towards an inclusion of that society within global structures. The 'globalisation' aspects of sociology are referred to as 'post-modernism' by some authors such as Moore (1966) and Featherstone (1985). Others, notably Giddens (1990), challenge the idea of post-modernity suggesting that modernity is the appropriate identification of present thinking. Whichever set of theorists make most sense to you, both parties recognise the development of the globalisation thesis, and both are interested, at least in the writings referred to, in the structural developments. These two sets of theories provide a current example of the dangers of classifying sociological theory and perspectives too rigidly.

For our purpose, the review of some key ideas that inform sociology, and the introduction of new terms such as modernity and post-modernity, are as far as a brief review of a theory can be taken. It is not necessary to pursue these terms in detail until you understand the basics of them; that would be essential if it was sociology as a science that you were studying. An awareness of those ideas current in sociology is useful when you are selecting from that science areas relevant in your journey to understand the social context of health and health care. In this way, you will be familiar with the terms and be able to place them as examples of the way in which some aspects of theory are presented in sociology.

Bear in mind, however, as you explore further into the arena of theory the words of Ian Craib (1984) who suggests that theory is 'necessarily fragmented and that we need different types of theory to explain different things'. Even within the notional grouping of 'structural perspectives' this sense of fragmentation becomes evident. At the centre of all structural studies is the 'reality' that society is an artefact, a construct which has been created. The focus for study varies depending on the perspective of the theorist, whose interests can vary from investigating the social functions of a major social institution, such as the family, to seeking to understand social evolution. You have read in the preceding chapters of the ways in which gender, age and 'race' are socially constructed. The researcher who is interested in, for example, age may have structuralist bias but may also be interested in the ways in which societal structures impinge on and are influenced by the individual.

Structuralism and Nursing

So far we have outlined some aspects of structuralism, and it would be reasonable at this point if the above were questioned as to its relevance to nursing and health care.

A brief reflection on the nature of a hospital will help you to recognise the structural relationships within the organisation of health care. The growing realisation of the impact of other nations and cultures on the development of health-care services lends some congruity for health workers to the globalisation thesis, and the need to take cognisance of such.

Changes and developments exist that indicate the influences of other parts of the world on the UK. Complementary medicine has increased in status, as we borrow from other cultures their traditional knowledge. Of course this is a two-way exchange and modern medical science is exported in turn, perhaps as vaccines and child-health knowledge. Not every exchange of knowledge is positive, and some of the impact of our own culture on the health of people in developing countries is in fact negative. The most famous example perhaps being the advertising of powdered baby milk within environments which lack the necessary clean drinking water and sterilising facilities to maintain the safe use of such products. It is pertinent to try to understand why impoverished mothers appear to be irrational in replacing free and hygienic breast milk for expensive and difficult-to-use powdered milk. Some understanding of the globalisation thesis and the impact of rich countries on the developing world is then one obvious route for study.

Reflection point 4.2

Consider for a moment what influences could encourage a mother to turn away from traditional ways of nurturing her baby, such as breast-feeding, and choose the more difficult and problem-laden route of bottle-feeding.

You could find it useful to think about some choice in your own life which seemed inappropriate to your family and friends.

Could similar pressures influence an individual's health decisions?

How does the developed world benefit from sales of powdered milk to the Third World?

Closer to home, an understanding of the nature of society contributes to the nurse's ability to provide comprehensive care. As will be seen later, policy decisions are linked to the nature of a society and subsequently have inevitable connections to the health-care services. To understand the nature of the these services and their relationship with other parts of society, the underlying structures that impinge on this arena need to be mined. A number of specialist texts are available which take a more in-depth approach to these wider issues in the sociology of health care. Gabe et al (1991) examine the current changes in the organisation of the health service, from privatisation to management and health-policy research. Jones (1994) combines an historical review of health and social policy with an analysis of the impact of such policy on some groups of individuals. Both these texts are presented in an elaborate academic style and are recommended for dipping into for key aspects of interest rather than to read in total, unless of course you find that you enjoy the writers' style and viewpoint.

Succeeding chapters will consider structural concerns like the re-organisation of the health service and developments in community care. Of major interest to any worker in the arena of health care is the link between poverty and health, and, again, later we will consider some major reports which are concerned with the consequences of low income and poor health. An examination of some of the causes of poverty will consider some of the structural explanations for differences in individual and specific groups' life chances. The study of populations and the emergence of population health research (Dean 1993) are promoting a resurgence of quantitative or positivistic approaches to research. These issues are examples of aspects of social life, relevant to nursing, which sit within the frame of reference of structuralist perspectives. In turn, you would be correct to think that such issues as poverty and health are as likely to have impact at a personal level as they are at a structural level. Key research box 4.1 indicates a key study that represents research strategies and interests from a structuralist perspective. The perspective or standpoint of interpretative approaches is more likely to be interested in the impact of structures on individuals and, further, to be concerned with the nature of that interaction, and the interaction between people. In sociological terms the word people would become 'social actors', something we will explore in the next section.

Interpretivism

This section examines some of the key elements of the interpretivist theory and the meanings that this could have for nursing and health care. As indicated above the interpretivist perspective is concerned with the

Key sociological research study: Structuralist

Durkheim 1970 Suicide: a study in sociology. Routledge and Kegan Paul, London

Durkheim's work was principally concerned with changes in the structure and stability of society. In 1897 he published what is now regarded as a famous study on suicide. He considered that social difficulties experienced by people in society created a sense of helplessness and isolation. As a consequence of such feelings, described by him as 'anomie', their social integrity was lost, enabling them to break the rules of society that forbade suicide. His hypothesis centres on the fact that social actions are attributable to significant social factors. In this study he found that suicide rates were higher in Protestant and lower in Catholic countries. He made links between the sense of 'anomie' experienced within a culture and the nature of the religious moral controls. He suggested that people from predominantly Catholic countries found more meaning in their lives and felt a sense of belonging that was not evident in Protestant countries; they were, thus, driven to the extremes of suicide infrequently.

His work has been criticised in recent times but remains one of the first analyses of the impact of society on the actions of the individual. His methodology is positivist and one key critic is Douglas (1974) who reviews Durkheim's work from a phenomenological perspective.

As population health research develops the major empirical studies like those carried out by Durkheim are beginning to find significance again. New methodologies are being developed to take into account the complexities evident in any attempt to study a society (Dean 1993).

**Reflection
point 4.3**

Unemployment, redundancy and homelessness are all aspects of life that impact on the individual in very specific ways. They may even be said to contribute to individual decisions such as suicide. Consider suicide, first, as a consequence of changes in the social order and, second, as a personal tragedy. Reflect on any significant differences indicated by these two interpretations of the cause of suicide. How may your own perspective influence your understanding of the needs of anyone who has tried to commit suicide but failed when they come into your care?

interpretation of the social world by social actors; that is the people who make up that world. As the structuralist perspective is concerned with structure, the uniting theme in the interpretivist domain is social action; that is the ways in which people act within social situations. Inherent in this viewpoint is the notion that people are social actors. The meaning of the word actor in this context is borrowed from the world of the theatre. As individual social actors move through the social world they assume a series of roles (Goffman 1969). These roles often have a sort of script, that is there are certain ways of acting defined as belonging within that role.

Reflection point 4.4	How many roles can you identify that exist in your own life?
	To what extent do you consider that there is a script for these roles. For example, is there some correct way to be a female aged 19 years seeking to become a nurse? Do men have to play a different role to present themselves as nurses?

If you think about the ways in which you act, within each of the various roles that are part of your routine life, you will find that some will have similarities whereas others are very different. The difference may be attributable to style of dress, demands of the actions you must take, language used, expectations placed on you and by you of others who share your various social experiences or roles. You may not have a script but you did learn the nuances of different role demands in some way. The interpretivist theorist in sociology is interested in understanding the nature of these many interactions.

As in structuralism, where several perspectives contribute to the theory building within that domain, this diversity is also evident within the interpretivist perspective. The dominant theories here stem from Weber, Schutz and phenomenology, Garfinkel and ethnomethodology, and symbolic interactionism.

Interaction is one of the key concepts which inform this perspective. Interaction may be a unifying factor, the common denominator that links these different theories as belonging under the one heading entitled 'Interpretivist'. Closer study of each of the areas reveals that real differences exist.

Ideal Types

Weberian theory emphasises the need to understand societal beliefs and the development of a reconstruction of the meanings given to the social world by individuals. He emphasised the need for society to be interpreted by the social researcher. A commonly-referred-to theme from the writings of Weber and other followers is the notion of the 'ideal type'. The work of Weber on such areas of social life as organisations and bureaucracy could possibly be seen as forming a bridge between the structural functionalists and the interpretivists. This would be a somewhat artificial link. However, it is tempting to contemplate the emergence of the study of society as providing a wider picture first, of structures and functions. Later developments move towards a greater understanding of the ways in which individuals experience the social world. The study of society combines an examination of the creation of society through interaction and the process by which meanings become attributed to events within a complex life experience.

This is a tempting overview, but it does compress some key differences that we need to explore. There are differences within interpretivist sociology that will become evident as frequently used terminology is explored. As outlined above, Weber presented the idea of the 'ideal type', which is a shorthand way of describing the significant elements of a phenomenon. These are not intended to be complete descriptions, just to provide a sketch of the main elements. This is perhaps almost a cartoon version of the phenomenon, in that it is the use of outline representation rather than detailed in-filling, which creates the image and makes it recognisable in other instances. You may have found references to ideal types of bureaucracy or to '**total institutions**'. Such references do not refer to the 'perfect' example, but to, for example, a psychiatric hospital as having the key elements that make up a 'total institution' (Goffman 1961). This is a particular aspect of social organisation that will be returned to later in this book.

Everyday Understandings

In contrast to the work of Weber, Schutz demands that the everyday understanding of the individual – rather than interpretations of the social observer – is of paramount importance. In the phenomenology of Schutz the notion of 'taken for granted' understandings of the world are important. Within this theoretical frame, social interaction is based on commonly held, shared, understandings of the social world. Theorists from this standpoint require that the methodology employed to investigate the social world will examine the shared understandings of the everyday world. Only in this way can the social observer seek to uncover the ideas and beliefs that guide and perhaps even direct individual action. At the core of such study is the intention to unwrap the processes of socialisation that enable us to internalise much of our social world. Linked to this is a requirement that the meanings that are explored are those of the social actor not the researcher.

In order to differentiate between the observations of the researcher or social observer, and the social actor, Schutz used the terms 'first and second order constructs'. A 'first order construct' is a way of identifying the commonsense understanding of the world as expressed by social actors.

When such expressions are gathered by the sociologist and used to create 'ideal types', these constructs, through the process of the development of ideas, have changed. The new theory that emerges developing an understanding of the first order constructs is presented in the academic language of the researcher and are referred to as 'second order constructs'. In this way the meanings of the social actors who are being studied, and those of the researcher carrying out the study, can be clearly differentiated. This is of central importance to the majority of interpretivists, who demand that any theory concerning the social world should examine the meanings attributed to social actions by social actors. This requirement, or rule, avoids glossing the meaning given to specific situations by social actors. The process of clarifying the meanings inherent in the language of the social actor discourages the overlaying of a theoretical language on to the everyday language.

Ethnomethodology

This refers to work of Garfinkel which was developed from that of Schutz. There are, therefore, some similarities, but **ethnomethodology** argues against the notion that all social actors hold similar assumptions so making interaction possible. Rather, according to writers such as Garfinkel, social actors have to work at each interaction. Ethnomethodologists are interested in the process of that 'work'. Maynard (1989:39) writes

> 'Ethnomethodology is concerned with the study of (-*ology*) ordinary people's (*ethno*) methods for making sense of and creating order in everyday life .... In general, ethnomethodologists try to avoid simply adopting the explanations and accounts of lay persons in their work. Rather, they take them as the *object* of their study.'

'Reflexivity' is a term associated with this frame of reference and is a way of stating that social actors create a situation by defining it. It is not possible to divorce actions from expressions of that action, that is talking about and doing are parts of the process of social construction. Conversational analysis has emerged from ethnomethodology and aims to build up an architecture of language through the study of everyday conversations. As individual social actors we take for granted the orderliness of talk. We have internalised the rules. The analyst seeks to understand the actual nature of these rules and so contribute to the wider study of conversation. The analysis of conversation is a valid activity and can be significant in health care. Major studies have been undertaken in relation to communication processes between nurses and patients. This research has contributed to changes in practice in relation to information giving (Fortin et al 1992, Gould 1990, Hayward 1975, Hiscock 1993).

Interaction

Yet a further division is evident in the work of the symbolic interaction-ists who, as might be taken from their title, find interaction to be central. It is the ability of humankind to interact, using and interpreting symbols, which makes us uniquely human and is central to the process of becom-ing social. Within this group of perspectives there are many divisions, per-haps the best known being the founding group, the Chicago School, which evolved as a response to the group's criticisms of functionalism. The symbolic interactionist seeks to understand the hidden meanings of the language and symbols that are part of interaction. Unlike the ethno-methodologist who views the social actor as being unconscious of the rules of interaction, the symbolic interactionist uses the structures of language to explore meaning.

One complication of both these perspectives is the nature of the sub-jects who form the focus of their studies. Both wish to delve into the hid-den meanings and understandings of the social world, and are concerned with the ways in which social actors interpret their world. Subsequently, there will be limited access to powerful and significant figures as a fea-ture of their studies. Much of the published work has centred on what could be regarded as non-typical situations, in particular the deviant indi-vidual became the focus for research (Becker 1966, Goffman 1961, 1970). Chapter 7 considers some of the key 'deviance' studies of particu-lar relevance to nursing.

Interpretivism and Nursing

Nursing is part of the social world. The meanings inherent in certain actions and interactions are as significant to nursing and health care as those noted in the wider social arena. Many texts on the sociology of nursing feature, as a focus, the relationships between the nurse, the doc-tor and the patient. These relationships are based on interactions, which each actor interprets and finds meaningful, whether at a conscious or unconscious level. In a later section this text will also consider profes-sional relationships and interactions.

The nature of patient-hood is of interest within this framework. You may have noted the way in which the status of patient is taken on board by people in an amazingly accepting way. Similarly, nurses are aware that some individuals seem easier to manage as patients: some are 'nicer' and more comfortable to work with than others. Studies in nursing which emphasise the need to seek the social actors' interpretation of their world are creating sources which can inform improved practice (Johnson & Webb 1995, Stockwell 1972).

Nursing practice has changed as more information on the needs of the patient or client emerges, demanding that nurses take into account more than their own interpretation of events. An awareness of the nature of the social world as a taken-for-granted entity has promoted extensive studies into the 'insider' world of the nurse and the patient. As studies are published, the rigidity of unchallenged traditions loses part of its tenacious hold on nursing practice. The nature of the patient–nurse relationship is examined in more depth in a later chapter.

It is tempting to view nursing as being one discreet role. On reflection, nursing can be seen as a series of roles, such as carer, manager, teacher, clinician, therapist, counsellor and so on. Even these roles can have sub-divisions; for example, caring can be divided into caring for and tending to. As you can now begin to see, by seeking to understand the various roles in nursing a wider picture can be achieved. The work of the nurse, with a taken-for-granted image of gentle hand on fevered brow, begins to be exposed as a more complex aspect of social interaction. It is of course a penalty of investigating the social actors' interpretations of events that some knowledge may be gleaned that is uncomfortable to take on board. Therefore, studies based within the interpretivist domain must take a 'warts and all' approach.

Discussion point 4.2

A number of key roles that the nurse takes in the care of the patient can be distinguished: carer, manager, teacher, clinician, therapist, counsellor.

Comment on the extent to which you consider these roles to be realistic.

Identify counterparts for these roles in other areas of social life.

Identify the aspects of such roles that would be of interest to an interpretivist.

Writings from the interactionist perspective frequently challenge the individual reader to question personal practice. Since the nature of this perspective is to unravel the nature and meanings of interaction it is possible to identify aspects of individual practice in theoretical explanations or descriptions. It is relatively recently that questions have been raised concerning the role of the nurse. The interpretivist theoretical stance enables the study of roles within nursing, providing a medium through which nursing practice can be improved at a personal and professional level.

Earlier in the chapter poverty was used to illustrate the relevance of the structuralism to nursing. Through interpretivist theory the realities and experiences of life in poverty for the individual patient/client are accessible. The nurse can both gain insights into the structures which contribute to the creation of poverty and the meanings of poverty for the individual and the nurse. Both groups of theory have relevance for nursing. It is common for individuals to have a bias towards one group.

Current writings on theory in sociology demonstrate that these two sets of theory, presented here as being in opposition, are more properly seen as being opposite ends of a continuum, but that nevertheless share much common ground. Theorists tend to move along that continuum rather than establishing fortified defences in one area. Essentially, the dominant perspective taken will be influenced by the subject of study and level of analysis, depending on whether it is the organisational or personal aspects that are to the fore of the research interest. Key research box 4.2 indicates a study that represents research strategies and interests from the interpretivist perspective.

Key research box 4.2	**Key sociological research study: Interpretivist** Becker HS 1966 Outsiders: studies in the sociology of deviance. Collier Macmillan, London Becker's work stems from the interactionist perspective and as the title of the selected study indicates his area of interest is the concept 'deviance'. His observations of marihuana users contributed to his theory concerning deviance. Unlike Durkheim, who considered deviance as rule breaking, Becker suggests that deviance is a label given to a rule breaker. In his study on marihuana use he identifies the social norms that create a sense of cohesion within the 'deviant' group and describes the sanctions imposed by the authorities to enforce social rules. The consequences of being labelled deviant can lead to exclusion from the dominant group. The deviant individual then takes up the new role and acts as expected. The labelling theory that emerges from much of this work has been influential in the arena of mental health where the stigmatising label of mental illness has been found to be detrimental to the individual. The work of Stockwell (1972) and others who have written about the unpopular patient have been influenced by labelling theorists.
Reflection point 4.5	In Accident & Emergency services there are often some patients who present difficulties because they bring with them social problems. Some of these problems are negatively labelled. Consider the descriptors 'drunk, tramp, para-suicide, confused'. Reflect on the ways in which these labels may affect the attitudes of reception staff and the care services that may be offered to people bearing such labels. To what extent do you think that professional people differentiate between patients based on socially ascribed labels?

Feminism

Before moving to the next section which is concerned with methods of investigation, this section offers a brief comment on one particular theoretical theme which is increasingly important in nursing and midwifery: **feminism**. For some this is almost a term of abuse to be used as some form of accusation for non-conforming staff. For others it is a central feature of working in a predominantly female environment which exists within a patriarchal society. Whatever personal bias is present, feminism cannot be overlooked.

Feminism emerged in the 1960s with the growth of the women's movement at that time. The focus of study has been to move beyond description of the social world towards seeking explanations as to why women are disadvantaged in relation to men. As was stated early in this chapter, the commonsense understandings of the social world are often taken for granted as 'truths'. Sociology demands that we review these assumptions, and sometimes offers surprises which are not always popular. This is particularly evident of feminist studies, and has significant impact for nursing, involving challenges to the accepted or taken-for-granted social order. In a society in which men have held power-based roles for so long that their positions have become regarded as 'natural', any form of study which threatens this viewpoint is unattractive.

As with the other two bands of theory, there is no single feminism. For each of the theoretical divisions there exists a corresponding feminist focus. Feminist writers have demonstrated that sociology has emulated the power structures in society and taken a predominantly male view. In the development of a feminist theory it is not enough to 'take women into account'. It is essential that the foundations of the theory start by taking into account female as well as male actions. There are feminist structuralists and interpretivists. Within feminist theory there are debates as to the relevance of the various perspectives, for example, the Marxist feminists are challenged by the materialist feminists. Maynard writes:

> 'Delphy's materialist model involves postulating the existence of two modes of production, the industrial and the domestic. In the industrial mode of production there is capitalist exploitation leading to the formation of two classes, proletariat and bourgeoisie. In the domestic mode of production there is patriarchal exploitation and the formation of two classes, men and women.'
> (Maynard 1989:64)

The one feature in common is that each perspective seeks to explain the oppression of women, and to take a female-oriented view of the social world. Feminists consider that sociological studies parallel the social world with regard to patriarchy. The studies which form the foundations of much sociological theory are biased towards male perspectives and have overlooked the female other than as domestic servants. Writers within feminist literature seek to move the female half of the social population from an implicit to an explicit presence in the theoretical analyses of the social world. Since the majority of nurses are women, feminist studies should be of critical importance. It is from the feminist writings that challenges to the contradictory imbalance between female nurses and male managers (the predominant mix) are emerging.

Theory and Method

We have examined two sets of theory: structuralism and interpretivism. Each theory has been identified with a particular style of approach to the study of the social world. Little has been mentioned of the methods used by each set of theories. This final section considers some of the general strategies in relation to methods of study specific to structuralism, interpretivism and feminism. There are many introductory texts, which focus on methods of research, that will balance the brevity of this overview. There is not scope here to enter into the wider area of research methods.

Within research methods it is usual to distinguish between two principal methodological approaches: quantitative and qualitative. These two strands can sometimes be regarded as extremes and in opposition to each other. Hypothetically, the two methodological approaches can be placed at opposite ends of a continuum listing the most typical data-collection methods for each extreme. The reality is frequently less clear, as researchers will often borrow strategies from both methodologies. Observation and interview are strategies used by many researchers irrespective of the nature of their theory base. The nature of the observation will vary from non-participant at the quantitative end of the continuum and move towards participant observation within qualitative research. Each set of theorists may have a different approach to using the various methods. It is also likely that a combination of methods is used, for example interviews and documentary data may be used to support a participant observation-based study.

The reality is that much research is carried out in the middle of this continuum, with researchers having a bias towards one or another theoretical framework. It is common to find that quantitative research, which emphasises the scientific method approach, is used mainly by structuralists. A frequent occurrence is that a research design which follows the positivist traditions and uses a survey-style method may use an unstructured interview to examine some key issue which has evolved from the research study. In this way the value is demonstrated of combining the positivist and interpretivist strategies in seeking understanding of the social world. We cannot and should not consider the social world only through its structures or the individuals who create that work. Rather, we are interested in both the internal and external construction of society. The eternal question posed when considering theory and methodology is the extent to which society is a creation of we, its members, or whether we are created by society.

Qualitative research is commonly used by researchers who favour the interpretivist perspective. The emphasis within this domain is that social research cannot follow the same principles used in the study of inanimate objects. The social actor has something to say about his or her world. The reflexive nature of the subject and the researcher must be taken into consideration (Hammersley & Atkinson 1983). Both subject and researcher are engaged in interpreting the world, and this must be taken into account during the research act and when analysing research findings. Research according to the interpretivist perspective must occur in a natural setting using natural methods.

Of course this brief synopsis makes distinctions which are less clear cut than is implied here. Further reading on this subject is necessary; McNeil's (1989) book is both brief and precise and a good overall introductory text, with accessible further reading sections.

Summary   This chapter has provided an overview of key theoretical perspectives. It is recognised that theory can be complex and elastic rather than clear cut and concrete. To allow a more flexible approach two main divisions of theory were addressed: structuralism and interpretivism. Feminism, as a theoretical framework which has a growing influence in nursing and health care, was also included. Links have been made between these theoretical frames and nursing and health care. A brief indication of the way in which theory influences methodology ends the chapter.

Further Reading

Giddens A 1976 Capitalism and modern social theory. Cambridge University Press, Cambridge

This is a good source for insights on Marx, Weber and Durkheim.

Giddens A (ed) 1997 Sociology: introductory readings, Part 1. Polity Press, Cambridge

The sections entitled 'What is Sociology' and 'Part XVI: Theoretical Perspectives in Sociology' provide an accessible opportunity to read extracts from the works of original theorists.

Maynard M 1989 Sociological theory. Longman, London
   This is a useful and readable overview of key theoretical perspectives, although it may phase the novice reader. Her further reading section also indicates some useful sources for those who wish to go beyond the basics of theory.

Scambler G (ed) 1987 Sociological theory and medical sociology. Tavistock Publications, London
   This provides a more in-depth discussion of theorists who have influenced developments in sociology applied to medicine and health. This book provides the opportunity to read a more focused review of the work of theorists such as Goffman and Foucault. It is for the adventurous reader rather than the novice.

McNeil P 1989 Research methods. Routledge, London
   A short and accessible book which introduces a range of methods in a straightforward way, without minimising the theoretical links and the complexity of undertaking research. It is particularly useful as an introductory text for those who need to develop the skills of critiquing research early in their course of study.

References

Becker HS 1966 Outsiders: studies in the sociology of deviance. Collier Macmillan, London
Craib I 1984 Modern social theory: from Parsons to Habermas. Wheatsheaf, Brighton
Dean K (ed) 1993 Population health research linking theory and methods. Sage Publications, London
Douglas J 1974 The understanding of everyday life: towards the reconstruction of sociological knowledge. Routledge and Kegan Paul, London
Durkheim 1970 Suicide: a study in sociology. Routledge and Kegan Paul, London
Featherstone M 1985 The fate of modernity: an introduction. Theory Culture and Society 2(3)
Fortin J, Schwartz-Barcott D, Rossi S 1992 The postoperative pain experience: a description based on the McGill pain questionnaire. Clinical Nursing Research 1(3): 292–304
Gabe J, Calnan M, Bury M (eds) 1991 The sociology of the health service. Routledge, London
Giddens A 1990 The consequences of modernity. Stanford University Press, Stanford, CA
Giddens A (ed) 1997 Sociology: introductory readings, Part 1. Polity Press, Cambridge
Goffman E 1961 Asylums: essays on the social situation of mental patients and other inmates. Penguin, Harmondsworth
Goffman E 1969 Presentation of self in everday life. Penguin, Harmondsworth
Goffman E 1970 Stigma: notes on the management of spoiled identity. Penguin, Harmondsworth

Gould D 1990 Empathy: a review of the literature with suggestions for an alternative research strategy. Journal of Advanced Nursing 15(10): 1167–1174

Hammersley M, Atkinson P 1983 Ethnography: principles in practice. Routledge, London

Haralambos M 1980 Sociology themes and perspectives. Unwin Hyman, Slough

Hayward J 1975 Information: a prescription against pain. Royal College of Nursing, London

Hiscock M 1993 Complex reactions requiring empathy and knowledge. Professional Nurse 9(3): 158–160

Johnson M, Webb C (1995) Re-discovering unpopular patients: the concept of social judgement. Journal of Advanced Nursing 21: 466–475

Jones H 1994 Health and society in twentieth century Britain. Longman, London

McNeil P 1989 Research methods. Routledge, London

Maynard M 1989 Sociological theory. Longman, London

Merton RK 1968 Social theory and social structure. Free Press, New York

Moore WE 1966 Global sociology: the world as a singular system. American Journal of Sociology 71(5)

O'Donnell M 1992 A new introduction to sociology. Nelson, Walton on Thames

Scambler G (ed) 1987 Sociological theory and medical sociology. Tavistock Publications, London

Stockwell F 1972 The unpopular patient. Royal College of Nursing, London

INEQUALITIES IN HEALTH CARE

Key concepts

- Defining poverty
- Historical perspectives on poverty
- Reinterpretation of poverty
- Poverty in Britain
- Poverty and health care
- Social class and health
- The Welfare State
- Welfare rights
- Citizenship
- Universalism
- A changing population
- Primary and secondary deviance
- Labelling
- Stigma
- Total institutions

Section 2 is entitled 'Inequalities in Health Care' as it has become evident since the creation of the Welfare State and the National Health Service that some groups of people within our society are healthier than others. This leads to the existence of an apparent inequality in the health status and the health-care provisions for some groups of people. The significance of age, gender, social class and ethnicity or 'race' to health status is discussed. Questions are raised, although not always answered in a definitive way. Take, for example, the various explanations offered as to why inequalities in health exist at all, within a welfare state, which offers services to all people, irrespective of background, and mainly free of charge.

You will find reviewed the main and competing explanations for these inequalities. As to which is the correct one you will have to examine your own values and insights and decide as to which is the most persuasive. Chapter 5 focuses on poverty as an attribute of lifestyle and its impact on health and health care is considered. Linked to this are the ways in which certain groups within society appear to be disadvantaged due to age, gender and ethnicity, issues central to the theme of Chapter 6. Discussion of some social and health-policy issues is a necessary background for the work of nurses and other health-care workers.

Chapter 7 takes the reader into the somewhat more esoteric world of deviance; it links with the previous discussion on inequality, and reflects on the groups in our society who are stigmatised and as such may experience deficits in health care.

The concluding chapter in Section 2 will consider again the relevance of these concepts for nurses and health-care professionals; especially as, the majority of such workers, if asked, would insist that they treat all patients/clients equally. This section underpins much of Section 3 and informs some of the material in Section 4.

Poverty in Health Care

Ronnie Moore and Sam Porter

<table>
<tr><td>Key concepts</td><td>
■ Understanding poverty
■ Historical background to poverty
■ The extent of poverty in Britain
■ Poverty and inequalities in health
■ Poverty in health care
</td></tr>
</table>

This chapter deals with three major and related issues. The first part of the chapter examines the notion of **poverty**, attempting to describe what has been meant by the concept over the years. The next area that is covered is the relationship between poverty and inequalities in health. Here we discuss the evidence concerning whether or not being poor is bad for your health. Having examined the relationship between social inequalities and inequalities in health, the final issue discussed is the relationship between social inequalities and health care, in other words whether or not the poor get as good a deal as the rich from health-care institutions and professionals.

What is Poverty?

Poverty often conjures up vivid images of severe hardship and suffering, very often far removed from our own experiences. As a Western country, with all the trappings of wealth that such a position in the global economy entails, poverty in Britain does not seem such an immediate issue, when compared to the problems faced by people living in the developing world. As well as being an advanced industrial nation, Britain is a parliamentary democracy with a free education system and a national health service, and claims to provide equal employment opportunities for all.

However, this image of a welfare state, where opportunities and services are there for all citizens, does not reveal the whole picture of social life in Britain. Crucially, Britain always has been, and remains, a socially stratified society, where the distribution of wealth is highly unequal, and where private education and private health care are important resources for those who can afford them. These sorts of inequalities in income and the attendant inequalities in opportunity (sometimes called life chances) and health (what we might term health chances; Moore & Harrisson 1996) might lead us to question the degree to which poverty has been eradicated.

Defining Poverty

Although inequality in income does not necessarily mean that those at the bottom of the income ladder are suffering from poverty, there have been few examples of societies where this is not the case. It is certainly not the case in contemporary Britain. For those living in the lower socioeconomic bracket, with small financial incomes, daily living often involves a meagre and limited lifestyle. Nor is it simply a matter of not having enough money; poverty also involves living on the margins of society, without power or even a public voice to express concerns. Often, the poor are victimised and blamed for their own poverty. Poverty is about being excluded from the advantages and benefits which are considered normal for most people in society. It also has a profound influence on such things as diet, social activities, psychological well-being and access to amenities.

Although the effects of poverty may be great, it is not at all easy to say exactly what poverty is. There has never been agreement on the definition of poverty, often because interpretations have been influenced by political considerations. Differences in how it is recognised and conceptualised lead to different theories about poverty and to measures (or lack of measures) to alleviate its effects and to steer social policy. Because attitudes, theories and practical measures to deal with the effects of poverty hinge on how it is perceived, the way we define it is crucial.

Historical Background

Historical accounts of poverty are a useful starting point and are important in that they provide a benchmark for directing our contemporary understanding of 'poverty' and 'the poor'. Historically, the poor were categorised into different groups. These included categories such as vagrants, paupers, migrants, the sick, the old and the able-bodied poor. An important distinction arose between the 'deserving' and the 'undeserving' poor.

As early as 1531, an Act of Parliament officially differentiated between the 'able-bodied' vagrant and those vagrants that could not help being in the position that they were in because of disability or sickness (Kumar 1984). The able-bodied poor were identified as 'sturdy beggars', who were seen as not wanting to work for a living. They were regarded as a threat to the moral, religious and political order of the day. Begging, for example, was considered a threat to public order and legislation made slothfulness a crime punishable by flogging. However, there was some recognition that, in certain circumstances, the able-bodied might not be in a position to work. Thus, for example, another Act was passed in 1572 recognising some groups, such as redundant soldiers, as being genuinely unemployed, thus exempting them from the extreme penalties of the vagrancy laws.

Since the Elizabethan Poor Laws of 1597, official attitudes to the poor have been embodied in a whole series of Acts. Legislation reflected the general reluctance of Government to take responsibility for the poor and infirm. It was widely held that official actions to help the poor would simply encourage idleness and thus make matters worse. Relief from poverty was generally regarded as a matter for the family, sometimes with the assistance of the church. Rather than being seen as being related to the way society was organised, poverty was seen as an individual matter, due to personal misfortune, or to character or moral defect.

Although the Poor Law provided basic relief from hardship and deprivation, its primary purpose was not charitable, but to ensure that the poor were effectively managed. The legislation provided for a harsh system of public provision for the poor and destitute. The New Poor Act of 1834, together with the Poor Law Amendment Act of 1837, marked a new approach to poverty. The aim now was to solve the problem of the 'able-bodied' poor by forcing them into workhouses if they wished to obtain relief. It was these Acts which guided official attitudes towards the poor for the rest of the nineteenth century and beyond. By the middle of the nineteenth century, workhouses were widespread throughout Britain. One of the effects of the harshness of this legislation was that it encouraged workers and their families to become mobile in search of work. This meant that workers previously tied to the land gravitated towards the cities to gain work in the factories that emerged from the industrial revolution.

As we have seen, as far as official attitudes were concerned, poverty was linked to the pathology of the poor person, rather than to the social, political and economic environment in which that person lived. In other words, it was the individual rather than society that was seen as the cause of poverty. However, not everyone thought that way. For concerned observers such as Frederick Engels (1892) and Karl Marx, the problem lay in the social circumstances that the poor found themselves in. These circumstances were the result of the development of uncontrolled capitalism. Rather than solving the problem of poverty, in many ways the drift of poor workers to the areas where they could find factory work made matters worse. As industrialisation attracted people to the large urban areas, hardship and poverty became increasingly concentrated, with the industrial working class (or proletariat in Marx's terms) being exposed to poor working and living conditions, including overcrowding, bad diet and lack of sanitation.

It was not only Marx and Engels who found nineteenth century capitalism an abomination. Writers such as Dickens and social reformers such as Chadwick exposed the effects of urban life on the industrial poor. One of the most influential of these reformers was the founder of the Salvation Army, Charles Booth, whose 'Life and Labour of the People of London' (1889) provides a stark picture of what life was like. Booth showed that poverty, bad working conditions, low income and ill health were related. He based his definition of poverty on the point where income was not large enough to sustain physical health, otherwise known as the subsistence level. In Booth's account, poverty meant being in a constant state of want, having to struggle for the basics essential for survival. Developing Booth's work, Seebohm Rowntree (of confectionery fame) further examined the link between income and diet and attempted to determine the minimum intake of food required for the maintenance of physical efficiency. Thus, both of these social reformers attempted to identify a fixed point of income, beneath which it would not be possible for a person to live and work. This became known as the *absolute definition of poverty*, in that it regarded poverty as relating solely to the amount of income necessary for maintaining minimum health and efficiency. Although Booth and Rowntree were both humane and advanced for their times, such a definition was harsh in that those who had barely enough to live on, and whose whole income went into the bare necessities of survival, were not regarded as falling within the remit of poverty as long as they just about succeeded to keep body and soul together. That said, Booth and Rowntree were able to demonstrate that, even according to this very minimal definition, large numbers of people in Britain were living in poverty. The importance of Booth and Rowntree was that they provided an important starting point for the subsequent debate on the social and health consequences of poverty. By establishing measurable (albeit crude) levels of poverty and devising means whereby it could be defined and conceptualised, they stimulated public and academic debate, and spawned a broad body of literature on poverty and on the sociology of health and illness.

Activity 5.1   Consider why Booth and Rowntree's studies were important contributions to understanding poverty.

The Reinterpretation of Poverty

In recent years, the use of absolute definitions of poverty has been questioned, and is now largely regarded as inadequate, in that it deals solely with the most extreme forms of material deprivation, and the bare minimum required to function properly. This assumes that, apart from differing biological needs (such as the different calorific intake of men and women), all people's needs are the same, irrespective of when or where they live. As a result, it ignores important social and psychological factors that affect people's needs. Societies change over time, and at any one time there are many different types of society in the world. It has been argued by more recent commentators on poverty that this means that what poverty is seen to be will also change over time and space. For example, what is regarded as poverty in the developing world is considerably different from what is regarded as poverty in the West. In addition, people's apparent needs in the West have changed over time. Thus, no one in the nineteenth century would have felt 'hard done by' because they could not afford a television for the simple reason that there was no such thing. However, nowadays, television is seen as an almost essential part of life. At an even more basic level, it is not so long ago that there was no such thing as toothpaste or toilet roll, yet now these items are regarded as essential to the maintenance of personal hygiene. Absolute definitions of poverty cannot take account of the fact that people's requirements do not stay the same. However, such approaches continue to be highly influential in the formulation of official social policy in areas such as state benefit levels.

Notwithstanding the continued influence of absolute definitions of poverty, since the 1960s a number of commentators have sought to introduce a more flexible approach to the definition of poverty. Probably the most influential of these has been Peter Townsend, who since the 1950s has conducted a series of investigations into poverty in Britain. In his influential study, 'Poverty in the United Kingdom' (1979), Townsend argues that poverty, rather than being seen in absolute terms, should be defined in relation to the general standards of society at a given point in time. In other words, if a person cannot afford those things which are generally regarded as basic to everyday life, then they should be regarded as being in poverty. Similarly Mack and Lansley (1985) described poverty as having to live without those things which are regarded as necessities by most people in society. By using public opinion surveys, they were able to demonstrate that there was actually a public consensus as to what people regarded as necessities. The approaches of both Townsend, and Mack and Lansley involve what is called the *relative definition of poverty*, because it is defined in relation to the general standards of society.

Although many social policy academics may have attempted to broaden out the way we think about poverty, governments continue to have a great deal of influence over its definition. First, governments are able to make up their own definitions, and use them to decide the degree to which, and to whom, welfare payments should be made (or not made). Second, governments often attempt to influence the way poverty is generally talked about. Thus, for example, the term 'inequalities of health' was dropped by the British Conservative government of the 1990s, and replaced by the far less alarming term 'variations in health'. The word 'inequalities', by definition, indicates that we have an unequal society; by contrast, 'variations' carries no such implication, in that variations can be caused by a lot of things, such as poor lifestyle decisions.

Reflection point 5.1

Consider the following two quotations:

'Poverty, like beauty, lies in the eye of the beholder. Poverty is a value judgment; it is not something one can verify or demonstrate, except by inference or suggestion, even with a measure of error. To say who is poor is to use all sorts of value judgments.'
  (Orshansky M 1969 How poverty is measured. Monthly Labor Review, February:37; quoted in Townsend, 1979)

'Measuring poverty is an exercise in demarcation. Lines have to be drawn where none may be visible and they have to be made bold. Where one draws the line is itself a battlefield.'
  (Desai 1986:23)

Question: Why is poverty difficult to quantify?

The Rise of the Welfare State and the Discovery of Poverty

Traditionally, relief for the poor and infirm came from the church and from charity. Despite being forced to play an increasing role in such relief since the time of Elizabeth I, the formal role of the government remained limited until well into the twentieth century. This changed in the aftermath of the Second World War. The war was fought on the promise that there would be a better and fairer life for all when it was over. Poverty, ignorance and ill health began to be seen as social evils that should not be tolerated in a civilised society.

During the war, William Beveridge was asked to write a report setting out recommendations as to what was needed to be done to improve the health and welfare of British society. When it was published in 1942, it was an instant best seller, selling well over 600 000 copies. Although Beveridge was commissioned to look into the specific area of social security, he argued that reform in this area, providing a minimum income for all, would be only a partial solution to society's problems. As well as 'want' there were four other 'giants' that needed to be dealt with in a comprehensive social policy. These were 'disease', 'ignorance', 'squalor' and 'idleness'. To deal with these would entail reform of health-care policy, educational policy, housing policy and economic policy (to ensure full employment). Although Beveridge's recommendations were not implemented to the letter either by Churchill's wartime National Government, or by Atlee's post-war Labour government, the major influence of Beveridge was that he crystallised the agenda for the direction of social policy after the war. Accordingly, in relation to health, the National Health Service Act was passed in 1946, unifying health services and providing a universal service free to all at the point of need. On 5 July 1948, known as the 'appointed day', both the National Health Service (NHS) and the National Insurance Scheme (for unemployment benefit) came into being. There were similar reforms in other areas, such as the Education Act of 1944, which established for the first time a comprehensive and progressive educational system for all (Bruce 1961). What is interesting about the date of this Act is that it was passed by the National Government, headed by the Conservative, Winston Churchill. This reflects the fact that, although Conservatives were somewhat less enthusiastic about some aspects of the welfare state, most notably those surrounding social security, there was a large degree of consensus about the need for state intervention to ensure a decent quality of life for all.

The consensus about the importance of the welfare state survived (albeit somewhat battered and bruised) up until the late 1970s, when a Conservative government under Margaret Thatcher came into power. In the view of this government, there was a problem that people had come to rely far too heavily on the 'nanny' welfare state. According to Thatcherite doctrine, this meant that they no longer took responsibility for their own lives, expecting the state to do everything for them. Central to Thatcherism was the belief that people should be responsible for their own lives, and the state should only intervene when it was really necessary. Part of this doctrine involved the belief that health and illness were also matters of individual responsibility.

The change in government attitude was not simply a matter of the thinking-up of a new dogma. Dependency on the state had indeed been rising. This was largely the result of an expanding older population and a rise in unemployment since the economic crisis of 1973. With the economy weak, there was pressure on the state from businesses to reduce the amount that was drained off to the state to fund welfare provisions. As a response to the combined pressures of economic crisis and increasing demand for welfare, the Conservative government developed radical policies during the 1980s. These involved both cuts in the amounts spent by the state, and the privatisation of many areas where the state used to be responsible. During the 1990s, the Major government consolidated this approach.

The Conservative governments of the 1980s and 1990s justified their efforts to reduce the scope and influence of the welfare state on the grounds that the existence of such a state only encouraged people to become dependent on welfare. Their strategy was thus to discourage what was called a dependency culture. Instead of relying almost solely on the state to help those in need, there was now a far greater emphasis on charities and other voluntary agencies, and on informal care by private individuals, often family members.

As far as poverty was concerned, there were attempts, such as that by the Secretary of State for Social Security in 1989, John Moore, to claim that the economic success of Britain had eradicated absolute poverty and that relative poverty was simply just another term for inequality. For the Conservatives, inequality was regarded as something that was both inevitable and healthy for a society, in that if we were all equally wealthy there would be no encouragement for hard work, or reward for talent. This sort of approach has meant that the issues of poverty and inequality have tended to play second fiddle to other economic issues, such as the control of inflation.

In 1997 the newly elected Labour government approached things rather differently. Tessa Jowell, Minister for Public Health, returned to the Beveridge Report for her inspiration. The five 'giants' of 'want', 'idleness', 'squalor', 'ignorance' and 'disease' were once again under attack. She is reported as saying:

> 'We want to attack the underlying causes of ill health and break the cycle of social and economic deprivation and social exclusion. The new proposals will replace part of the Health of the Nation policy brought in by the Conservative government. This set out 29 targets to reduce the number of deaths from the biggest killers and causes of ill health. While many of these targets have already been achieved or are set to be achieved, the Government said Health of the Nation failed to look at the underlying reasons for ill health.'
> (Mihill 1997)

Her strategy represented new proposals for targeting poverty, unemployment, bad housing, social isolation, pollution, ethnic minority status and issues surrounding gender.

| **Discussion point 5.1.** | Discuss the notion that relative poverty is just another term for inequality. |

The Changing Population

As was noted in the previous section, one of the pressures on welfare state budgets is the increasing numbers of older people in the population. This process of **demographic change** has been going on for over a century, although it has recently accelerated. It is a result of the combination of a general decline in the birth rate and an increase in life expectancy. Since the start of this century, the percentage of the population over retirement age has increased from 8% to 21%. By the early 1990s, one in 14 of the population were aged 75 or over (Scambler 1991).

A key factor in this process has been a general improvement in the health of the population. Infectious diseases such as cholera and tuberculosis, which were once major killers in the West, have now largely been controlled (although the latter disease is making a worrying comeback). As McKeown (1979) points out, much of the decline in mortality from infectious diseases was a result of improvements in diet, living conditions and sanitary environment, along with the increasing availability of contraception which enabled women to control the number of offspring. The technical capacity to control fertility has been reinforced by the weakening of religious control and the changing expectations of women.

All these factors, in combination with technical and medical innovations, and the ability of people to access these improvements following the foundation of the National Health Service, have led to a considerable improvement in survival rates. This, in turn has led to an increasing number of elderly people, who, having completed their working lives, are often dependent on state pensions for their income. As the value of state pensions fall in relation to the income that other people enjoy, and as health services, which older people use more than younger, are cut back, the health and welfare of older people comes increasingly under threat.

From the above we can see that, ironically, the relationship between poverty and health is not all one-way traffic, in that part of the reason for there being a large group of older poor people is because the population has, in general, become more healthy and therefore survived longer.

The Extent of Poverty in Britain

Having examined successive British governments' attitudes to the issue of poverty, we now need to look at the evidence which indicates whether or not poverty has become less of a problem.

It has to be said that most evidence points in precisely the opposite direction. For example, Wilkinson (1995) notes that the poorest 10% of the population have seen their incomes decrease in real terms over the previous decade. He argues that this has had a significant impact on the

lives of children and young people, and warns that the long-term consequences of this decrease in the wealth of the poorest are yet to be realised.

Similarly, Jane Millar (1993), following a comprehensive review of
statistics concerning the *income poverty line* (the point of income below
which people are regarded as being in poverty), concluded that poverty
rates had risen substantially in the past decade. (The review included
analysis of statistics from the Department of Social Security, the House of
Commons Social Security Committee, and from the independent
'Breadline Britain' surveys.) Millar states:

> 'whatever measure of poverty is used, the picture is clear: poverty is wide-
> spread in this country, affecting about 12 to 13 million people, with about
> three to four million living in severe poverty. People of working age, and
> their children make up the majority of those living in poverty.'
> (Millar 1993:14).

Some might object to the suggestion that what has happened in Britain
is simply the result of a global economic downturn, which has affected all
countries, that have been forced to cut back on welfare expenditure in
order to keep budgets in line with national income. However, such an
interpretation has been challenged by Oppenheim & Harker (1996), who
argue that the growing divide between rich and poor in Britain is almost
unique in international terms.

> 'Between 1979 and 1992/3 the real incomes (after housing costs) of those
> in the poorest tenth fell by 18 per cent; the average rose by 37 per cent,
> while the richest enjoyed a staggering rise of 61 per cent. In international
> terms, the UK experienced the sharpest rise in inequality, with the excep-
> tion of New Zealand, according to the Joseph Rowntree Foundation Inquiry
> into Income and Wealth.'
> (Oppenheim & Harker 1996:1–2)

It should also be noted that poverty and deprivation are unevenly spread,
with some regions, towns, communities and ethnic groups experiencing
greater concentrations of deprivation than others (Blakemore & Boneham
1994, Evason 1985).

Poverty and Inequalities in Health

Having indicated that poverty remains a problem, the next thing we
need to do is to track the relationship between poverty and ill health. The
first thing to note is that in Britain, as in other advanced Western nations,
we have seen a marked improvement in the overall health of the
population. However, although this may be the case in general terms,

there is increasing evidence indicating that improvements in health are directly linked to one's position in society. Favourable health appears to be associated with wealth, whereas ill health is disproportionately distributed among the poor and those who are socially deprived.

It is not easy to establish definitively the relationship between poverty and health. Much of the difficulty comes from problems of definition. We have already noted how difficult it is to pin down the concept of poverty. There are similar problems with defining health. Like poverty, there is no fully agreed concept of health or illness. Rather, these concepts are interpreted differently in different social, political and cultural contexts (Blaxter 1990, Blaxter & Paterson 1982, Herzlich 1973). The World Health Organisation has recognised this difficulty, and now only claims to provide 'working definitions' of these concepts.

Because this issue is difficult does not mean that we can say nothing about the relationship between poverty and ill health. There is considerable evidence that they are linked. Much of the data providing this evidence was initially gathered by the Research Working Group on Inequalities of Health in the 1970s. The Working Group was commissioned by the Labour government of the day, because of increasing concerns that 30 years of health care by the National Health Service did not seem to have resulted in the sort of improvements in the health of the poor that health care which was free at the point of delivery was expected to make. It was the task of the working group to analyse the extent and causes of variations in health between members of different occupational social classes.

The findings of this working group were published in what is popularly known as the Black Report (DHSS 1980). The findings of the Black Report confirmed widespread class differences in health, and argued that reduction of those differences was beyond the scope of the NHS on its own. Indeed, the report noted that since the inauguration of the NHS, the health gap between the rich and poor had widened. Whereas those in the lower economic class levels were indeed healthier in the 1970s, their rate of improvement was far less than those in the higher occupational class levels.

An array of socioeconomic factors, such as unemployment, lack of transport, education and environment were cited in the Black Report as influencing health. The common denominator relating to all these factors was occupational social class. The Black Report recommended that wide-ranging social reform, which would deal with the issues such as poverty, social deprivation, diet, and housing and working conditions, was needed if the standard of health in Britain was to be significantly raised.

Since the publication of the Black Report, official and independent statistics from a variety of sources have revealed clear mortality trends related to social class (Marmot & McDowall 1986). However, by the time the report was published, there was a Conservative government in office, and its main recommendations were never implemented. Nevertheless, the report did have a profound impact, in that it stimulated research on poverty, social inequality and health on both a national and international level. To a large extent, this body of research evidence supports the main findings of the Black Report and its identification of a link between poverty and ill health.

Indeed, since the publication of the Black Report, there is evidence that things are getting worse rather than better. For example, a further report, 'The Health Divide' by Whitehead (1987), commissioned by the Health Education Council, suggested that health inequalities were widening during the 1980s. This conclusion has been reinforced by other researchers, such as Phillimore et al (1994), whose study of Northern England showed considerable and widening disparities in mortality rates between affluent and deprived areas. This rather depressing scenario of a country riven with health inequalities was summed up in the 1994 NCH Action for Children report:

> 'In Britain today low income groups consistently show higher rates of all the major killer diseases. Lower income groups also experience higher rates of chronic sickness and their children tend to have lower birth weight, shorter stature, and other indicators suggesting poor health status. The unemployed and their families have considerably worse physical and mental health than those in work.'
> (NCH Action for Children 1994:1)

This survey showed that one in five parents had gone hungry in the previous month because they had no money to buy food for themselves. One in ten children under five had gone without food in the last month because there was not enough money. The survey also demonstrated that the food the poor did buy was not very nutritional. This was explained in terms of cost. The cost difference between a healthy and an unhealthy shopping basket per week was on average £5. Although this may not seem very much, it constituted one fifth of the total weekly expenditure on food of families living on Income Support. The survey found that it was lack of money rather than ignorance that led to poor diet. Parents' perceptions about the quality of their families' diets was generally accurate: 'families are aware of good eating practice but their budgets did not allow them to put this knowledge into practice' (NCH Action for Children 1994:17).

Explanations for Inequalities in Health

It would seem by this stage that it is clear that there is a link between poverty and ill-health. However, this is not the whole story. So far, we have only identified what is technically called a correlation, that is we have observed that the two things go together. What we have not identified is a causal relationship: we do not know why they go together, and more specifically, we do not know if poverty and inequality cause ill-health, or whether the relationship between the two is caused by something else entirely. This issue has been at the centre of debate, with a number of competing explanations being posited.

The first explanation to be considered is known as the 'artefact' explanation. This involves the assertion that the relationship between social inequality and differential health chances has been created by the researchers (an artefact being something made by people). In other words, the argument is that these findings have more to do with the process of explaining the relationship than with the actual relationship itself. Much of the debate here involves rather technical statistical arguments, relating to how statistics are derived, compiled, manipulated and interpreted (see, for example, Bloor et al 1987). One example of this sort of critique is Klein's (1988) argument that it is impossible to state with any degree of certainty that inequalities in health are widening over time. This is because the social classes being examined have themselves changed in size and composition over time. This means that longitudinal comparisons of class statistics do not compare like with like. Klein has also asserted that the Black Report's exclusive concentration on statistics pertaining to the working population means that the picture it painted was far gloomier than was really warranted. This was because it did not take into account that sector of the population that had enjoyed the greatest increases in life expectancy, namely those over retirement age. These sort of objections carry some weight, although they qualify rather than refute the central arguments. As we have already noted, the concepts of poverty and health are extremely difficult to pin down and therefore equally difficult to measure. As such, critiques like those above are important because they provide a means of improving future research design.

Another objection to the argument that poverty causes ill-health is that this is to put the causal relationship the wrong way round; in fact, it is ill-health that causes poverty. This sort of argument has its roots in sociological interpretations of the work of Charles Darwin, in that it sees natural and social processes as a form of a selection of the fittest. Basically, the argument is that differences in the general health status of different occupational social classes is the result of selective social mobility. It is argued that there is a tendency for fitter and healthier people to move up the social ladder, and for sicker people to drift downwards. Thus, although such an argument does not deny that class inequalities of health exist, it asserts that this is simply because good health will tend to improve your socioeconomic status, while ill-health will disadvantage you (Stern 1983). Once again, there is probably some truth to this argument.

A final objection accepts that there is a link between poverty and ill-health, but argues that the link lies in the behaviour and attitudes of the poor. This argument is linked with what is known as the 'culture of poverty' thesis (Lewis 1961, Murray 1989), which argues that the poor have a self-destructive culture, which leads them to act in ways that are bad for their health. In other words, the poor tend to become ill because of the lifestyles and personal habits in which they engage. To put it crudely, the poor tend to get sick not because they are poor, but because they smoke too much, drink too much alcohol, fail to take exercise and eat the wrong sorts of food. Probably the most famous example of this approach was the attack made by former Conservative minister, Edwina Curry, on the diet of those living in northern England, which she blamed for making people of that area less healthy, on average, than their southern counterparts.

In one way, this argument has a degree of truth to it. In another way, it is difficult to understand, in that this issue was dealt with in the Black Report and 'The Health Divide', with the latter going to considerable lengths to ascertain the degree to which lifestyle factors led to inequalities in health. The reports did not seek to deny that 'the evidence . . . suggests that differences in life-style could indeed account for some of the class differential in health' (Townsend et al 1992:323). However, they went on to point out that, although lifestyle differences between the occupational social classes could account for some of the differences in health, they could not account for them all. They noted that there were a number of convincing studies designed to control for (that is take account of the effects of) lifestyle factors which still demonstrated inequalities in health. One of the most famous of these was the Whitehall study (Marmot et al 1984), which followed the health of over 17 000 civil servants since 1967. In line with the 'culture of poverty' thesis, Marmot et al discovered considerable differences in the average lifestyle of members of different civil service grades. Thus, for example, whereas only 29% of the 'top' grade smoked, 61% of the 'bottom' grade were smokers. It is not hard to see how this difference would have an effect on the relative health of both groups. However, taking one disease that is closely associated with smoking, coronary artery disease – and controlling for smoking, systolic blood pressure, plasma cholesterol, height and blood sugar – the study discovered that the risk associated with employment grade was reduced by just a quarter.

In contrast to these explanations, there remains the materialist interpretation that argues that health is directly affected by the material circumstances in which people live. For those living in poverty, housing circumstances, diet and leisure, for example, are all curtailed by the material deprivation that they experience. It is not simply a matter of those living in poverty making different choices because of their culture, rather that they have little choice about how they live because their position in society means that they do not have the wherewithal to make choices that would improve their health chances. In short, the health of a person is closely related to his or her social circumstances (Power 1994).

To take the built environment as an example, spores from mould in damp housing have been shown to cause respiratory disease (McCarthy et al 1985). Bad housing, including architecture, design, construction and insulation have been shown to be detrimental to health. Lowry (1990) has shown how cutting back on building costs and the use of poisonous materials, such as asbestos, lead to chronic ill-health. Ironically, the costs cut on building are passed on to the National Health Service in the form of costs for medication and hospitalisation because of the chronic illness that results. The character of poorer areas is also said to be damaging to health. McIntyre et al (1993) argue that living in more affluent areas means better access to quality foodstuffs, better recreational facilities and public services. Conversely, the Glasgow Healthy City Project (1992) noted that poorer areas tended to have poorer outlets for quality food. When this is combined with difficulties in transport, either due to cost or the absence of public transport, it means that people living in these areas have little access to the sort of foodstuff that constitutes a healthy diet. The significance of not being able to access a healthy diet has been underlined by Barker et al (1988), who noted that children from unemployed households tended to be shorter in stature than those from households in which a parent is working.

Case study 5.1

Six-year-old Daniel lives with his parents in a poorly maintained, very damp flat on the sixth floor of an inner-city tenement building. Daniel suffers from bronchitis and asthma but his parents do not have the financial resources to afford a more suitable living environment. To all intents and purposes this family are in a poverty trap.

What action can health professionals take to help families such as this improve their quality of life?

Access to heat is another very important material factor, affecting most acutely the young and the old. In relation to this issue, provisions for the poor in Britain are especially bad in international terms. Allamby (1987) has argued that whereas other European countries with climactic conditions similar to, or better than, Britain have comprehensive plans to alleviate the effects of extreme weather conditions, Britain does not. These policies include regulations to ensure high building standards in relation to insulation, and energy and health-care policies which are geared to the needs of the vulnerable population. Britain does have policies of this sort, including the cold-weather payments scheme, but these are far less generously funded or effective than their European counterparts. As a consequence, Britain has higher morbidity rates in vulnerable populations than comparative countries in Europe. Moreover, Allamby argues that the problem is almost certainly underestimated because its real extent is unknown. This is largely because hypothermia is rarely given as the cause of death. Allamby notes that there is a linear increase in cerebral and coronary thrombosis as the temperature decreases and argues that this indicates a connection that should be taken into account when measuring the health costs of lack of access to warmth.

Poverty in Health Care

Having examined how poverty relates to health chances, we now discuss how it relates to health care. Research suggests that the poor do not have equal access to the full range of health-care facilities, and that they under-utilise health-care resources. This has been known for a considerable time. For example, Titmuss (1958) demonstrated major differences in the utilisation of health-care services in the period after the inauguration of the National Health Service, with those in the higher income bracket better able to access services, and most notably specialist care. Hart (1971) noted that the geographical location of health-care services tended to be inversely related to the needs of the population. Deprived areas, where people had greater need of health care because of the relationship between poverty and health, had fewer health-care resources, with health-care services being concentrated in more affluent areas, where needs were less. Moreover, there is evidence of differences in treatment when people do seek health care. Cartwright & O'Brien (1976) and Blaxter (1984) have argued that the quality of interaction and the time afforded to working class patients in medical consultations is inferior to that given to middle class patients.

The problem of access to health care was highlighted by a Dispatches Report (Yates 1995) on Channel Four television, entitled 'Serving Two Masters'. This report by John Yates illustrated a two-tier system of health care. One of the problems he identified was the fact that medical consultants were allowed to work for both the National Health Service and the private sector, with little control over the amount of work they did in the latter sector. This practice consistently disadvantaged the poor, who, having no choice but to depend on NHS provisions, were forced to wait for long periods of time before they received treatment.

The report showed that surgeons in two of the specialities with the longest waiting lists spent, on average, one and a half days per week treating private patients.

'The waiting times in the public and private sector are starkly different ... It is difficult even to put the two sets of figures on the same scale ... Of private patients, 96 per cent see a consultant in under a month, but in the NHS only 9 per cent have such an option. In the private sector, the waiting time of most people is 21 days or less – in the NHS, some will have to wait 21 months! We have a health-care system which, for both out-patient consultations and operation, now treats the rich more quickly than the poor.'

(Yates 1995:5)

In 1978, at the Alma Ata Convention, member states of the European region of the World Health Organization made a commitment to improve the general health of member nations. Part of this commitment was to strive for equality in health care by the year 2000. The British Government's response to this commitment is outlined in the 'Health of the Nation' (DoH 1991). Although the rhetoric in this document promotes the objective of equity in health care, the subsequent evidence indicates that this is not happening. Indeed, with recent reforms of the NHS, which have promoted the influence of market principles, there is a danger that inequalities in access to health care will increase further.

Activity 5.2   Try to discover what your local health targets are and see how these relate to World Health Organization aspirations for Health for All.

Summary   This chapter has considered poverty, health and health care as separate but closely related issues. It has looked at historical attitudes to the poor and outlined absolute and relative definitions of poverty. The extent of poverty in Britain has also been outlined. We have also discussed major demographic changes over the past century, as these have had a direct bearing on the poverty and health debate. Inequalities in health have been discussed, along with explanations for these inequalities. Finally, we have examined the link between poverty and health care.

Further Reading

Griffiths S 1994 Poverty on your doorstep. London Borough of Newham Poverty File
   This profile draws together statistical and other data which identifies the nature of deprivation in one of the most deprived inner-city areas in Britain.

Kempson E, Bryson A, Rawlingson K 1994 Hard times. Policy Studies Institute, London
This is a report of a Joseph Rowntree Foundation research project containing reflections on the lives of 74 families living on very low incomes. Trying to 'make ends meet' is at the heart of this book.

Oppenheim C, Harker L 1996 Poverty: the facts, 3rd edn. Child Poverty Action Group, London
This book explores the key components of poverty. Factors such as unemployment, debt, regional, national and European dimensions of poverty are discussed, as are the experiences of women and minority ethnic groups. This book does not claim to offer in any detail the range of possible solutions to poverty but offers insights as to its cause.

References

Allamby L 1987 Dying of cold: fuel poverty and ill-health in Northern Ireland. Northern Ireland Council for Voluntary Action, Belfast

Barker M, McLean S, McKenna P, Reid N, Strain J, Thompson K, Williamson A, Wright M 1988 Diet, lifestyle and health in Northern Ireland: a report to the Health Promotion Trust. University of Ulster, Coleraine

Blakemore K, Boneham M 1994 Age, race and ethnicity: a comparative approach. Open University Press, Buckingham

Blaxter M 1984 Equity and consultation rates in general practice. British Medical Journal 288: 1963–1967

Blaxter M 1990 Health and lifestyles. Routledge, London

Blaxter M, Paterson L 1982 Mothers and daughters: a three-generational study of health attitudes and health behaviour. Heinemann, London

Bloor M, Sampier M, Prior L 1987 Artifact explanations of inequalities in health: an assessment of the evidence. Sociology of Health and Illness 9: 231–264

Booth C 1889 Life and labour of the people of London. Williams and Norgate, London

Bruce M 1961 The coming of the Welfare State. Batsford, London

Cartwright A, O'Brien M 1976 Social class variations in health care and in the nature of general practitioner consultations. In: Stacey M (ed) The sociology of the NHS. Sociological Review Monograph 22. University of Keele, Keele

Department of Health (DoH) 1991 Health of the Nation. Department of Health, London

Department of Health and Social Security (DHSS) 1980 Inequalities in health: report of the Research Working Group chaired by Sir Douglas Black. DHSS, London

Desai M 1986 Excluding the poor. In: Oppenheim C, Harker L (eds) Poverty: the facts, 3rd edn. Child Poverty Action London, p. 23

Engels F 1892(1993) The condition of the working class in England. Oxford University Press, Oxford

Evason E 1985 On the edge: a study of poverty and long-term unemployment in Northern Ireland. Child Poverty Action, London

George M 1993 Nursing Standard 7(49): 21–23

Glasgow Healthy City Project 1992 Food, poverty and health, Conference proceedings, cited in George 1993

Hart J 1971 The inverse care law. Lancet i: 405–412

Herzlich C 1973 Health and illness. Academic Press, London

Klein R 1988 Acceptable inequalities. In: Collinson P, Green D (eds) Acceptable inequalities? Essays on the pursuit of equality in health care. Institute of Economic Affairs, London

Kumar K 1984 Unemployment as a problem in the development of industrial societies: the English experience. Sociological Review 32(2): 187–208

Lewis O 1961 The children of Sanchez. Random House, New York

Lowry S 1990 Getting things done. British Medical Journal 300: 390–392

McCarthy P, Byrne D, Harrisson S, Keithley J 1985 Respiratory conditions: effects of housing and other factors. Journal of Epidemiology and Community Health 39: 15–19

McIntyre S, MacIver S, Sooman A 1993 Area, class and health: should we be focusing on places or people? Journal of Social Policy 22(2): 213–234

McKeown T 1979 The role of medicine. Basil Blackwell, Oxford

Mack J, Lansley S 1985 Poor Britain. Allen and Unwin, London

Marmot M, McDowall M 1986 Mortality decline and widening social inequalities. Lancet ii: 274–276

Marmot M, Shipley M, Rose G 1984 Inequalities in death specific explanations of a general pattern? Lancet 1003–1006

Millar J 1993 The continuing trend in rising poverty. In: Sinfield A (ed) Poverty, inequality and justice. New Waverley Papers, Social Policy Series No 6, Edinburgh

Mihill C 1997 Ministers launch crusade to upgrade public health. The Guardian, 8 July, p 5

Moore R, Harrisson S 1996 In poor health: socio-economic status and health chances. Social Sciences in Health 1(4): 221–235

Murray C 1989 Underclass. Sunday Times Magazine, 26 November: 46

NCH Action for Children 1994 Poverty and nutrition survey. NCH Action for Children, London

Oppenheim C, Harker L 1996 Poverty: the facts, 3rd edn. Child Poverty Action, London

Phillimore P, Beattie A, Townsend P 1994 Widening inequality of health in Northern England 1981–1991. British Medical Journal 308: 1125–1128

Power C 1994 Health and social inequality in Europe. British Medical Journal 308: 1153–1156

Scambler G (ed) 1991 Sociology as applied to medicine. Baillière Tindall, London

Stern J 1983 Social mobility and the interpretation of social class mortality differentials. Journal of Social Policy 12: 27–49

Titmuss R 1958 Essays on social welfare. Allen and Unwin, London

Townsend P 1979 Poverty in the United Kingdom. Penguin, London

Townsend P, Davidson N, Whitehead M 1992 Inequalities of health: the Black Report and the Health Divide. Penguin, Harmondsworth

Whitehead M 1987 The health divide: inequalities in health in the 1980s. Health Education Council, London

Wilkinson R 1995 Unfair shares: the effects of widening income differentials on the welfare of the young: a report for Barnardo's. University of Sussex, Brighton

Yates J 1995 Serving two masters: consultants, the National Health Service and private medicine. Dispatches Report for Channel Four television, London

6 Disadvantaged Groups in Health Care

Sandra Ryan

Key concepts
- Universalism and citizenship
- Individual differences in health care
- Citizenship and health care
- Institutional factors affecting disadvantaged groups
- Unemployment and low-paid work

This chapter is concerned with the individual and institutional factors which impinge on access to health and welfare for some groups in our society. It begins by describing the development of citizenship and explores the problems faced by disadvantaged groups in securing citizens' rights in the provision of welfare. It argues that, despite assertions by policy makers, that the present model of welfare is targeted in order to meet those most in need, there is a common purpose across all disadvantaged groups which should unite all citizens in a re-affirmation of the idea of universal rights for all.

Universalism in access to welfare has been the subject of debate since the beginning of the welfare state in 1948. However, in recent years the idea of universal rights to health and wealth has been clouded by the many social changes that have taken place including a change in political ideology, the economics of Western capitalism and the changing nature of debate in social theory.

One of the increasingly popular theories is postmodernism with its key ideas of individualism, diversity and choice. Parallel to this theoretical development, the political ideology informing policy – in this instance health policy – centres around individualism and consumerism, within a market-led economy. The rationale behind the change in welfare provision is based on more choice for individual citizens. The idea of 'citizenship' in the context of various charters has re-emerged as part of government policy. Central to this is the idea of 'consumer sovereignty' with promises to respect individual choice in a range of services from education to health care. Within nursing this is reflected in new styles of nursing care designed to promote individually tailored care, under the labels of the nursing process and more recently primary nursing under the 'named nurse' policy. It has been argued that nursing has become:

> 'Non standard and non mass produced. It is highly individualised, highly differentiated and, through negotiation with the client, is totally responsive to consumer demands.'
> (Gough 1994:261)

The moves towards individualism in government policies, social theory and nursing care are not without cost. They may cloud the many disadvantages which are shared by different social groups. This in turn will encourage social planning and health-care provision to move further away from equal and universal access.

Universalism and Citizenship

Welfare 'reform' of the past three decades replaced the notion of universal rights to state welfare with one of private welfare for those who can afford it. An example of this is the development of private insurance and pensions, with only minimal state provision for those not privately covered. This change in policy will have a profound effect on the quality of living for those who are excluded from participating in the free market including: women, because of their over-representation in part-time low-paid and informal labour; the Black populations, because of discrimination in access to secure well paid employment; and those who already rely on diminishing state provision, because they too are excluded from the private markets, namely disabled people and the older population (Alcock 1989:32).

One of the problems with the argument in favour of universalism is that it has been shown to advantage the more articulate middle classes both through employment within the welfare services and through a greater use of services by the better off (LeGrand 1982). Alcock argues that the biggest problem in state provision has been the domination by professionals and bureaucrats who have targeted services with little or no input by service users themselves. He suggests that this lack of consumer consultation has been exploited by previous Conservative governments who used the idea of consumer sovereignty to mislead clients into thinking they had some control over the provision of services (Alcock 1989). One of the ways in which this process has manifested has been in the re-emergence of the idea of citizenship as part of government policy.

Individual Differences in Health Care

Citizenship: The Theory of TH Marshall

The early 1980s witnessed a revival of the notion of citizenship as a means of securing universal rights, including health and welfare, for all citizens of Britain. This development emerged against a background of a powerful state which increasingly regulates our lives in both the public and the private domains (Taylor 1989). Although the notion of citizenship has a long history, recent debates can be traced back to the theory of citizenship developed by Marshall in the 1950s. Marshall's model consisted of three elements: civil, political and social.

> 'The civil element is composed of the rights necessary for individual freedom – liberty of the person, freedom of speech, thought and faith, the right to own property and to conclude valid contracts, and the right to justice . . . . By a political element I mean the right to participate in the exercise of political power, as a member of a body invested with political authority or as an elector of the members of such a body. . . . By the social element I mean the the whole range from the right to a modicum of economic welfare and security to the right to share to the full in the social heritage and to live the life of a civilised being according to the standards prevailing in the society. *The institutions most closely connected with it are the educational system and the social services.*'
> (Marshall 1950:10) (Author's italics)

Marshall's theory of the development of citizenship has been criticised from many different angles by social commentators in different camps. Marshall himself acknowledged the paradox that the growth of citizenship – which is concerned with equality – has coincided with the development of capitalism (Mishra 1977). Other critiques of Marshall's work point to: its Anglo-centrism, that is it concentrates on the idea of being British (Mann 1987); its inability to recognise that there are different interpretations of what citizenship means to different people rather than a single definition (Turner 1990); and the neglect of the 'public/private' space arguments, i.e. the autonomy of the individual in the private sphere as distinct from state regulation in the public (Turner 1990). Yet others have argued that these critiques concentrate exclusively on class and neglect issues of gender, ethnicity and physical ability, which exclude many members of society from participating as full citizens with equal political and social rights. Although accepting the underlying positive side of citizenship, Walby notes:

> 'Today citizenship means universalistic democratic rights of social and political participation. In popular political discourse it entails the full

integration of all adults regardless of 'race', ethnicity, sex or creed. In this way it is a modernist, universalistic concept. However, it is also a national project, a location which places limitations on its universalism .... Access to citizenship is a highly gendered and ethnically structured process.'
   (Walby 1994:391)

So far the discussion about citizenship has been limited to an abstract description of its origins as a concept and the arguments which point to the complexities of attempting to attain universal rights for all citizens. It is necessary to have a brief historical perspective before evaluating the concept in relation to health and access to health care. Citizenship has been discussed by social commentators, primarily as a right, from a 'bottom-up' approach. More recently, in what may be seen as a 'top-down' approach, citizenship has entered the language of government policies.

Citizenship and Health Care

Following the health service reforms which started under the Thatcher-led Conservative government in the early 1980s, a different notion of citizenship began to emerge. Part of this new approach was the emergence of citizens' charters which came about alongside changes to a market economy in the provision of health and welfare services. There is a mirror image here of Marshall's observation that the evolution of citizenship has occurred alongside the development of capitalism. Health service provision has become resource-led to the extent that services have changed beyond recognition from the 1948 'cradle to grave' promises. What has emerged is a mixed economy where those who can afford it are encouraged to turn to private health care rather than depend on state provision. Alongside this, the Conservative notion of citizenship is loaded with responsibilities as well as rights. However, it is unclear how beneficial the part of the equation relating to rights is to many groups in our society. For example, this version of citizenship relies heavily on individual responsibility for health; in some cases this could be construed as 'victim' blaming. An example of this is the idea of 'unhealthy lifestyles' which cites acts such as smoking or alcohol abuse as causative factors while ignoring underlying socioeconomic determinants of ill-health such as unemployment, poverty and poor housing (see Chapter 5 for a fuller discussion of these points).
   Part of the 'top-down' approach to citizenship was the introduction of citizens' charters, including the Patients' Charter (DHSS 1992), which set certain efficiency targets to be met by health authorities. These targets covered a range of areas from out-patient waiting times to dealing with complaints. However, it has become apparent that the charter does not have any great effect on the quality of service provision. For example,

reduction of out-patient waiting times has served only to exert pressure on health service staff who must increase patient through-put which in turn means that patients have less time with clinical staff on their hospital out-patient visits.

The Patients' Charter (DHSS 1992) promised the following.

- Respect for privacy, dignity and religious and cultural beliefs will be afforded to everyone.
- Arrangements will be made to ensure everyone, including people with special needs, can use services.
- Arrangements will be in place to ensure that relatives and friends can receive information about the progress of a patient's treatment, subject to the patient's wishes.
- Following a 999 call an emergency ambulance should arrive within 14 minutes if you live in an urban area, or 19 minutes if you live in a rural area.
- Upon being taken to an accident and emergency department a patient will be seen immediately and the need for treatment assessed.
- Individual patients will have a named qualified nurse, midwife or health visitor to care for them.
- Before discharge from hospital a decision should be made about any continuing health-care or social-care needs the patient may have. Arrangements for meeting these needs will be agreed between the hospital and agencies such as community nursing services or local authority social services departments. With the patient's agreement, carers will be consulted and informed at all stages of the process.

Activity 6.1   Consider the contents of the Patients' Charter. When you have read the chapter, return to the charter and discuss how many of the points will have an effect on the disadvantaged groups' access to welfare. Write an alternative charter.

As we will see below, the health service reforms have yet to have any real effect on those members of society who were disadvantaged in their experiences of health care prior to reforms and remain so following them. The rights and responsibilities of citizenship are effected by age, ethnicity and gender. These individual factors will now be considered in turn.

Age

Older people in our society are one of the groups who are labelled as causing the greatest drain on resources, particularly health resources (Ham 1992). Indeed, in health service debates older people are discussed using the most negative terminology; they are a drain on resources, a burden to families and health service providers, and a high-cost user group of health services. As in most industrial societies, the population of older people in Britain is increasing. However, despite the negativity directed towards the older population and their use of health services, it is important to note that the majority of this group care for themselves in their own homes (Neave 1994). Not only do they care for themselves but many also care for dependent spouses, and some for their own children who may be young adults with long-term disabilities (Parker 1992). They also make a major contribution to the informal economy by their participation in voluntary groups, often providing services which arguably should be provided by the state (Neave 1994). So where does this leave the older population in relation to their rights as citizens? As we have already discussed, citizenship carries with it rights as well as responsibilities. It could be argued that those who were able have fulfilled their responsibilities over the years, by contributing to the economy in both a formal and informal way. A society which values its older people would acknowledge their lifetime contribution in fulfilling their responsibilities and would meet their needs as they become less able to contribute to the economy. Unfortunately this is not the case. The lack of value directed at a large population of citizens is notable in the provision of health care which both stereotypes and patronises the older population. There is a long history of poor funding to the 'Cinderella services' for the older population and the chronically ill. This has been reinforced by a medical model of care which emphasises a curative approach to health care and actively directs funding towards 'high tech' expensive care such as cardiac surgery and intensive care. This style of care concentrates efforts at the younger, economically active population, at a cost to service provision for residential care and community care for the older and chronically ill (Ham 1992).

Under the Conservative administration of the 1980s and 1990s health service policy changed dramatically from one of 'provider' of services to 'enabler' within a competitive market environment. Services would be purchased within the public, private and voluntary sectors. The rapid change to market forces left members of the older population at a disadvantage. Those who were able to pay for services were expected to do so, while others could be forced to sell the family home to pay for private residential accommodation. However, the most vulnerable older people, those who had never been in the position to save and plan for their old age, would be forced to rely on their families and poorly financed state services. Walker (1987) argues:

> The "dependency" of many elderly people and its severity consist of a structurally inferior social and economic status in relation to the working

population and, secondly, that social policies sponsored, directly or indirectly, by the state occupy a role in the creation and management of that dependency.'

(Walker 1987:41)

Economic policies are reinforced by ageist attitudes towards the older population by those working in and managing the health services. Cornwell (1989) argues that such attitudes are expressed at both individual and structural levels within the NHS. Neave (1994) notes the effect that this discrimination has on the lives of older people:

'Stereotyping ... assumes an extra importance because it influences the way the defined group perceives itself. If an older person accepts that they have less worth than younger members of society, and are a burden, they do not articulate their needs and ageism persists. Moreover, they are often less able, because of frailty, to press for change.'

(Neave 1994:199)

Cornwell's assertion that dependency is reinforced by the ageist attitudes of health workers themselves should alert nurses to consider there own culpability in perpetuating **ageism**. Nurses work most closely with those in need of health care in the community and in hospitals. It should become the responsibility of nurses to work with and support the older population in their attempts to change the stereotype of the 'no-longer economically viable dependent'. This project could start by working in partnership with older people and challenging ageism in health-care contexts. This may seem a very small step in the face of the unremitting tide of capitalism; however, changing ageist attitudes of health service personnel is a start in securing support for this section of the population who have met their responsibilities as citizens all of their lives and should continue to enjoy the rights of citizenship in their later years.

Case study 6.1	Consider the following situation:
	An 80-year-old woman living alone has recently become wheelchair-bound due to arthritis. Before this she was independent and cared for herself at home. Both her GP and family are trying to persuade her to sell her home in order to pay for residential care. She is adamant that she wants to stay at home.
	Which agencies (if any) should be involved in the 'case management' of this woman? Where do you see a nursing role in helping to fight the paternalism and dependency inherent in the proposed option of care?

'Ethnicity'

Chapter 5 gave details of the Black Report (DHSS 1980) and the Health Divide (Whitehead 1987) which indicated that people of ethnic minorities are highly represented in groups which suffer low-paid work, unemployment and poverty, all of which are related to ill-health. Consequently these members of our population suffer higher rates of mortality and morbidity. Research to date appears to have concentrated on those conditions which are confined to specific ethnic groups, for example thalassaemia and sickle cell disease. Maslin-Prothero (1994) indicates that there is a wealth of evidence to suggest that these areas have been researched by white researchers out of interest, rather than in response to the wishes of the affected population (Donovan 1986, Pearson 1986, Torkington 1987, Williams 1989). In fact those conditions which are of most concern to discreet ethnic groups are in fact the same as the population in general; for example: respiratory disorders, infertility, psychosexual problems, allergies and diabetes. The available research on ethnic-specific illnesses covertly implies 'victim blaming', that is, the cause of ill-health is culturally and racially connected.

Access to 'ethnically appropriate' health services in Britain is affected by both overt and covert discriminatory practices based on racism. Covert (or hidden) racist practices by some health authorities may be among the reasons for members of different ethnic groups suffering through lack of services. One such example of covert racism is the lack of comprehensive screening for blood disorders such as thalassaemia and sickle cell; another is the inappropriate care of the Asian population who suffer high incidences of osteomalacia and rickets. To explain, despite pressure from campaigning groups there is still no routine screening for those who may carry or suffer from sickle cell anaemia and thalassaemia, or adequate resources for effective treatment (McNaught 1987). This is despite the fact that sickle cell anaemia is found in 1 in every 200 Caribbean births and 1 in 100 West African births (Thomas-Hope 1992). Maslin-Prothero points to the discriminatory practice of the routine screening for all babies in Britain for phenylketonuria, a rare disorder only affecting Caucasians, which occurs in only 1 out of 10 000 births (Smart 1987, Thomas-Hope 1992). The other example of discrimination in health-care provision is the refusal of the British government to allow those foods in regular use by the Asian population to be fortified with vitamin D, which has successfully reduced the incidence of rickets in the non-Asian population through the addition of the vitamin to margarine (Grimsley & Bhatt 1988, Torkington 1987). The previous Conservative government's alternative strategy of issuing a health directive to the Asian population to expose their skin to more sunlight in order to help the body's production of vitamin D was equally culturally insensitive in that it failed to take into account the important cultural and religious implications for Asian women who expose very little of their skin.

Reflection point 6.1

Maslin-Prothero (1994) has suggested a change in the nursing curriculum in order to insure that nursing care is culturally appropriate. Think of some examples where a patient's cultural beliefs may cause conflict in an in-patient enviroment. How would you ensure that culturally appropriate care was part of your work?

Returning to the issue of citizenship with the expectation of each individual's right to equality and respect within British society, certain ethnic groups in Britain are indeed disadvantaged. One of the counterarguments, mentioned briefly earlier, is the notion that citizenship is based on ideas of 'nationhood'. That is, the acceptance that all citizens within Britain experience equal respect and access to public services, such as health care. However, the Anglo-centric argument put forward by Taylor and others, combined with the history of Britain's colonial past, has profound implications for some members of the population, and can be examined in relation to the Black populations of Britain. Indeed the health service itself is one institution which in times of economic regeneration relied on immigrant labour from colonies and former colonies to carry out work that was deemed beneath the employable population of Britain of the time. Yet in times of economic hardship such immigrant labour is vilified for taking jobs that could employ white males. Many migrant labour forces do not gain full citizenship in the country to which they travel for employment. This is one of the factors that continues to militate against some members of the population gaining full citizenship, with associated rights. Many members of the population have only partial subject status, that is, they are only entitled to partial rights as citizens of Britain. In terms of health expectations we have already mentioned the evidence from the Black Report and the Health Divide which indicate the connections between unemployment, poverty and ill-health, and that members of 'ethnic minorities' are heavily represented in these groups and there-

Reflection point 6.2

The population of Britain are subjects in a constitutional monarchy rather than citizens within a constitutional framework. Many immigrant workers gain partial subject status for different periods of time and some are deported following their use as part of the labour force.

What does this tell you about the nature of 'citizenship' in Britain today? Consider the health implications of such an insecure existence on a family that has travelled to Britain to work.

fore suffer higher morbidity and mortality rates than the wider population in British society.

Disability

It is fair to say that a great deal has been done in recent years to raise the profile of the needs of disabled people in the media. Much of this work has been carried out by disabled people themselves, tired of the imagery of helpless members of society who rely on sympathy and state aid. However, although disabled people themselves have become organised in fighting for equal treatment as citizens, a great deal of change in public attitude and government policy is still required.

The language and theoretical perspectives associated with studies of **disability** varied greatly over the latter half of the twentieth century. Much recent debate has focused on the political correctness of terminology. Words like 'mentally retarded' and 'spastic' are no longer socially acceptable and quite rightly so. It is essential that offensive terminology is removed from our language and that particular groups decide which terms are the most appropriate. However, simply changing terminology, without changing discriminatory practices does not provide equality for disadvantaged groups.

There are historical and economic factors which determine how disability is classified and viewed in different societies. In advanced industrial societies the prevalence of disability is related to an increase in the population of the very old, advances in medical care of premature babies, and an increase in machinery and road traffic accidents. By contrast, in developing countries disability may be caused by poor nutrition in pregnancy and early life, lack of adequate health care, and the effects of war and hostilities. A widespread example of the latter cause can be seen in the land mine injuries suffered by civilians in South-East Asia.

Oliver (1990) suggests several definitions of disability. The first is the notion of punishment: a family with a member with a disability may view it as a punishment from God or nature depending on their beliefs. Second is the notion of 'liminal' existence, that is, disabled people are neither sick nor well but existing in a kind of 'limbo' on the margins of society. Yet another ominous suggestion is that of 'a surplus population' theory, this has been a policy in times of economic need in developing countries (resulting for example in widespread infanticide) and also as a political ideology such as that espoused by Fascist Germany during the holocaust years of the Second World War. Oliver (1990) suggests that the dominant view in Britain today is the 'personal tragedy' theory. In this case disabled people are viewed with philanthropy and pity. Oliver uses the term 'social oppression' to describe discriminatory practices against people with disabilities. He began his arguments by noting that in his own subject area, sociology, academic studies of disability were few, echoing the same marginalising effect of disability in society. Social oppression theory suggests that those in society who are not disabled maintain (for their own advantage) the hierarchical nature of a society, which views disabled people as inferior. Townsend & Davidson (1992) confirm the empirical evidence to support this conclusion. Because we live in a capitalist society and disabled people often cannot make the economic contribution expected of all citizens, they are particularly disadvantaged in terms of employment, education, housing and transport. It is important to consider the term 'social oppression' throughout this chapter when we note that more than half the people who are disabled also suffer discrimination on the basis of gender and ethnic origin (Oliver 1990).

Disabled people are disadvantaged in health terms in a variety of ways. The medical model of care, which has taken upon itself the responsibility of classifying disability, has an unprecedented amount of power in affecting life chances of a disabled person. It has a direct influence on a disabled person's right to be employed, to claim unemployment benefit on the grounds of being unfit for work, and in determining the style of education open to that person (Oliver 1990). The medical model also concentrates on curative medicine, with an emphasis on 'normality' in relation to health. This does not take into account the social abilities of disabled people which would allow them to participate more fully in the workforce and in education if they were not 'labelled' by health professionals as being other than 'normal' (see Chapter 7 for a full discussion on labelling). The medical dominance in decision making for disabled people, particularly those in institutions, has had a profound effect on the poor quality of their lives. One of the more positive changes in health care provision is that following the Community Care Act (1990); a case manager, in many cases a social worker, is the professional responsible for organising care packages based on individual need. Although far from establishing full citizen's rights for disabled people, in that provisions are dependent on resources available, the Community Care Act goes a small way towards involving the person who has the need in planning his or her care.

Reflection point 6.3
Pause to consider the role that nurses have played in maintaining a dependency culture for people with disabilities.

How can nurses redress this situation?

Gender

Gender is of central significance when discussing socially oppressed groups in all spheres of life. The organisation of health-care services to date has done little to promote women-centered care, indeed the organisation of welfare services as a whole has followed a model of care which places women in a position of dependency on men and the state. In short women's health is affected by the domination of patriarchy in everyday life and a male medical model of health care provision.

Doyal (1995) has argued that the way women's health is viewed (in global terms) is problematic in that it is still dominated by a medical model of care which concentrates on the biological functions and dysfunction of the body, treating the body as a piece of machinery that can be 'fixed'. She claims that in order to understand women's health, organisers of health policy and care should examine the social circumstances that pertain in their lives which directly affect health, rather than concentrating so much on disease-oriented epidemiology. Her crosscultural analysis of women's health chances concentrates on women's labour and the household economy, marriage and marital status, motherhood, the hazards of domestic labour, and poverty. Doyal notes that 'despite cultural variation between communities, it is usually women who continue to be expected to take responsibility for what is regarded as 'domestic work' (Doyal 1995:28). There is a growing body of feminist literature in sociology and social policy which emphasises the oppression of women whether in social policies (Pascall 1986, Williams 1989) or in the masculinisation of everyday life (Davies 1995, Walby 1990). For almost two decades critics of the organisation of welfare, who also have a renewed interest in citizenship, point to the continued emphasis of a woman's place being within the family despite the changing nature of women's work outside the home and the changed nature of the family itself. Describing the effect of the daily grind of domestic labour on women's health Doyal asserts:

> 'The most obvious characteristics of domestic work in all countries are probably its open-endedness and its sheer volume. There is no limit to how much can be required in any given period, and no entitlement to holidays or even meal breaks. Very importantly there may be no obvious end to the working day, so that many may find it difficult to separate work from rest or "leisure". Indeed those with young children may never really be "off duty" as working hours even extend to periods of snatched sleep. For many this can lead to a punishing burden of both physical and mental labour.'
> (Doyal 1995:28)

Despite the years of intensive campaigning and consciousness-raising by those interested in gaining equal status for women, many health and welfare policies are still organised on the assumption that a woman's place is in the home. One stark illustration of this in terms of health care changes was the Community Care Act (1990) which relied on the continuation of care for dependents to be carried out in the home, predominantly by women with little or no support (Parker 1992). Evidence from the Black Report and the Health Divide shows that women are highly represented in all of the disadvantaged groups, with the corresponding implications for ill-health. The majority of women who live on or below the poverty line are older women dependent on state benefits or young women caring for small children alone (Graham 1993, Popay & Jones 1990).

Returning to the question of citizenship with its associated rights and responsibilities, it appears that women are disenfranchised because of the low value placed on care work at home and the fact that national insurance contributions and pension schemes leave women dependent on men and/or the state. Like the population of older people, women have rather more responsibilities than rights.

Socially Oppressed Groups

There is disagreement among social scientists about the ways forward for equality of health for all and whether or not this is an appropriate or achievable goal. Oliver's (1990) assertion that disabled people are a socially oppressed group is equally valid when examining other disadvantaged groups such as women, older people and those of ethnic minorities. One of the thorny issues in discourse regarding disadvantaged groups in health care is that of social class. Disagreements range between a Conservative assertion that we now have a classless society, on one extreme, to the Marxist, or 'political economy', view that we live in a society highly segregated by class and the ability of individuals to contribute to the capitalist economy.

Social Class and Health

Social class is the area most frequently visited in the 'individual' versus 'structural' debate, in relation to inequalities in health and health chances. There is clear evidence to suggest that patterns of ill health and death are closely related to social class (Nettleton 1995). For example data from the Office of Population Censuses and Surveys (OPCS 1986, 1988) indicates the following.

- Compared to babies born to parents in Social Class 1, babies born to parents in Social Class 5 are almost twice as likely to be stillborn or die in the first year of life.
- Men in Social Class 5 have a 2.4 times higher mortality rate than those in Social Class 1.

Other methods of measuring health indicators yield similar data, for example:

- Men in Social Classes 1 and 2 are 1.5 times more likely to report their health as 'good' or 'very good' than those in Social Classes 4 and 5.
- Both men and women in Social Classes 4 and 5 are four times more likely to report their health as 'bad' or 'very bad' than those in Social Classes 1 and 2. (White et al 1993)

Reflection point 6.4

Consider for a moment the above bulleted points. Reviewing the information about an individual group's disadvantages in health, do you think that nurses and other health-care workers can discount a class analysis of inequitable distribution of wealth and access to quality health care? What are the arguments for and against class analysis? (You will need to refer to Chapter 2 as well as the information here.) Where would you place the occupation of nursing in a class analysis of professions?

Institutional Factors Affecting Disadvantaged Groups

It is difficult to untangle all of the factors which affect different disadvantaged groups in their experiences of health and wealth. However, there are clearly three facets of our society which oppress all the individual groups, namely sexism, racism and capitalism. This section focuses briefly on the following institutional factors:

- access to health care
- institutional racism
- unemployment and low-paid work
- housing and health.

Access to Health Care

The proposed reasoning behind the move towards consumerism in health care in recent health service reforms was to raise the standards of care, allow patients more freedom of choice about the type of care they wish to receive, monitor quality of service provision taking into account consumers' views, and give access to a complaints procedure for customers unhappy with their experiences of care. As was mentioned earlier, this 'customer care' was enshrined in the publication of the Patients' Charter (DHSS 1992). This emphasised the government's shift to the individual rather than a collective right to good health care for all. Over time, it has become apparent that the Patients' Charter is more a public-relations exercise than addressing real health inequalities. Consumerism has been described as a gloss, a 'supermarket' model, which allows people the choice whether or not to accept the goods on offer but does not allow any access to decision making or the more fundamental aspects of control over health-care provision.

One illustration of this was the change in the structure of provision of care at general practice level. The rhetoric behind the supposed aim 'to give patients . . . better health care and greater choice of the services available'(DHSS 1992:3) was belied by the fact that it is the purchaser, for example the fundholding GPs, who make decisions about where care is purchased, rather than the consumer. Once a GP has made a contract with a particular provider of service, it is very difficult for a patient to seek his or her care elsewhere (Walker 1993). This also places a strain on GPs who soon realise that their elderly and chronically ill patients are costly to care for and therefore unattractive prospects to have on their books. So it seems that the move to 'consumer-led' care may lead to discrimination and poor access to quality care for certain 'unattractive' groups of patients.

Institutional Racism

Racism in our society is inextricably linked with Britain's colonial history. In the immediate post-war years when the labour pool was diminished, people from British colonies and former colonies were actively encouraged to come to Britain to fulfil those jobs that others deemed unpalatable or too low paid. Today, people from 'ethnic minorities' are still over-represented in those occupations connected with hazardous factory work, domestic work and other low-paid occupations where shift work and poor working conditions prevail (Nettleton 1995). The 1991 census revealed that this section of the population is more likely to live in areas that are materially deprived. In such materially deprived areas they experience discrimination in housing applications which results in overcrowding – another factor associated with ill-health. Material deprivation is, as we know, also linked to ill-health. This lack of secure employment opportunities maintains material deprivation for people from ethnic minorities, who are poorly represented in the better paid jobs, particularly the professions. Where they are in such professional groups they are rarely in positions of authority and power (Campling 1994). In short, a significant number of people in Britain experience institutional racism in the search for employment, in maintaining secure employment, in attaining adequate housing, and in their experiences of education – all factors which influence health (Blackburn 1991).

We need look no further than our own profession, nursing, to see how institutional racism affects those employed in the National Health Service. One of the institutions which actively sought employees from abroad in the early 1950s was the health service. Many of those who chose nursing entered into the 'less prestigious' areas, such as the care of older people, those with mental health problems and those with learning disabilities. Moreover, they were also employed in the lower echelons of the nursing hierarchy; for example, the Equal Opportunities Commission noted in 1991 that black recruits were often not informed about SRN training at the time of recruitment. NHS managers have perpetuated the erroneous belief that black nurses are more suited to 'bedside' nursing because this is what they prefer. Baxter (1988) suggests that the lack of such nurses entering the 'widened' selection process for nurse training is the result of two factors. The first is their experiences of discrimination on application, and the second is that family members who have worked in the health service relate their own negative experiences and discourage their application. Maslin-Prothero (1994) suggests that the nursing curriculum itself needs to change along with the initiation of active recruitment policies for ethnic minorities. She asserts:

'If nursing is to reflect the UK's diverse population and provide appropriate care, we must address issues regarding race and equality of opportunity in recruitment and selection procedures. If the black populations are not represented in nursing, and especially in positions of power where decisions are made, the needs of the black population are not ultimately going to be addressed and met.'
(Maslin-Prothero 1994:186)

Case study 6.2

Saiid has been a Staff Nurse for over 10 years. He has undertaken postregistration education and management training courses in his field of nursing. However, during a recent internal trawl and subsequent interview for a charge-nurse post he was turned down in favour of a more junior member of staff with less experience who was white.

Consider for a moment your own area of work. Have you or a colleague experienced racism, in overt or covert form? Or, in looking more widely than your immediate colleagues, who holds the positions of power in your organisation? Thinking carefully and honestly, do you think racism exists in your place of work? If you were a nurse manager, how would you address this situation if it is the case?

Unemployment and Low-Paid Work

The Black Report and the Health Divide showed that there is a strong connection with unemployment, low-paid work and poor health. There has been a sustained ideology in Britain's welfare provision of categorising those who are materially deprived into two camps: the 'deserving' and 'undeserving' poor (Ditch 1987). The unemployed, particularly the long-term unemployed, fall into the latter category. Postwar governments have consistently tried to reduce wage bills at the same time as lowering the amount and range of benefits in order to 'price the unemployed into jobs' (Ditch 1987:33). There has been a persistent but false perpetuation of the myth that the long-term unemployed do not want to work. This stigma has marginalised this group of the population who are forced to live on inadequate benefits and who are the least likely to vote in parliamentary and local elections and thereby exert no influence over policies affecting their lives. It is difficult to imagine how the long-term unemployed can exercise either their rights or their responsibilities as citizens when they have no control over their circumstances and can do little to change them.

Housing and Health

Since the 1930s there has been a dramatic improvement in housing standards in Britain which should have had a direct effect on the quality of life and therefore health. Nonethless, inequalities in housing provision and the consequences of poor housing on health are still a major concern in the 1990s. In 1987 Wicks noted that the measurement of housing quality was hampered by a lack of adequate statistics but that those that were available revealed massive inequalities. Adequate space, ventilation, heating and clean water are all essential amenities and have a direct effect on health. The consequences of poor housing such as chronic illness,

Reflection point 6.5

What are health implications of the following factors?

■ A consultation paper by the Department of Environment (DoE) which suggests that homeless families should no longer have priority for permanent housing.

■ A survey of young people in Birmingham by Barnardos which showed that one in four were either living in hostels, had been offered places in hostels or were sleeping rough. Four out of ten were homeless.

■ A report by the Joseph Rowntree Foundation which found that 1.64 million properties still fail to meet the basic standards of fitness laid down by the DoE.

■ One in four house buyers who bought between 1988 and 1991 hold properties worth less than their mortgage.

■ House buyers of this era in serious arrears are falling into homelessness and bankruptcy because of failures of insurance protection services and social security.

(Source: Campling 1994)

depression, infectious diseases and family breakdown have been well documented over many years. In the 1980s the Conservative government introduced a home ownership policy to actively encourage council tenants to become owner-occupiers. However, the house-purchasing boom of the 1980s followed by recession has left many citizens in serious economic difficulties and added to the numbers of homeless (Campling 1994).

Summary   This chapter has given a brief overview of some of the issues which cause certain groups in our society to be disadvantaged in terms of access to health care. The ideas of citizenship and consumerism, enshrined in successive government policies, have yet to have any real effect on the lives of many members of our society. Some commentators would argue that the climate of individualism in policies and in social theory in the late 1990s cloud the real issue of the increasing inequalities in welfare provision in Britain (Taylor-Gooby 1991, Williams 1992). Nursing, too, has become seduced by the emphasis on individualism and choice. It is time for nurses and nurse theorists to step back and examine this trend, taking into account our role as formal carers in an ever-diminishing welfare state. One way of achieving this is to become active citizens and join in the welfare right's movement in campaigning for universal health care for all, regardless of status. As Alcock notes:

'Perhaps the most important potential strength which welfare rights and citizenship offer a future campaign of state welfare is the renewal in them of an appeal for universal values and universal rights. The social rights of citizenship unite those whom the market inevitably divides. They also provide a base for unity of purpose across the divisions class, race, and gender. All citizens have basic needs in common, the need for health, for education, for shelter, and (in cash economy) the need for a sufficient income.'
(Alcock 1989:37)

Further Reading

Glendinning C, Millar J (eds) 1992 Women & Poverty in Britain in the 1990s. Harvester Wheatsheaf, New York, London
This book contains chapters on women, age, family and welfare issues that consider the disadvantages over time and class for women and their families living in poverty. The sections are clearly defined and will provide a valuable extension of your reading.

Widgery D 1992 Some lives! A GP's East End. Sinclair-Stevenson, London

In contrast to Glendinning and Millar's academic prose this book is part social commentary and part personal reflection on the life of a GP in East London. The varied lives of the people he visits and the often direct circumstances in which they live are presented with humanity and humour. These observations of a professional person, battling against the odds of social inequalities, makes powerful and interesting reading.

References

Alcock P 1989 Why citizenship and welfare rights offer new hope for welfare in Britain. Critical Social Policy 9: 32–43

Baxter C 1988 The black nurse: an endangered species. National Extension College, Cambridge

Blackburn C 1991 Poverty and health: working with families. Open University Press, Buckingham

Campling J 1994 Social policy digest. Journal of Social Policy 23(4)

Cornwell J 1989 The consumers' view: elderly people and community health services. Kings Fund, London

DHSS 1980 The Black report. HMSO, London

DHSS 1989 Caring for people. HMSO, London

DHSS 1992 The Patients' Charter. HMSO, London

Davies C 1995 The professional predicament in nursing. Open University Press, Basingstoke

Ditch J 1987 The undeserving poor: unemployed people then and now. In: Loney M (ed) The state of the market? politics and welfare in contemporary Britain. Sage, London

Donovan J 1986 Black peoples' health: a different approach. In: Rathwell T, Phillips D (eds) Health race and ethnicity. Croom Helm, London

Doyal L 1995 What makes women sick? Gender and the political economy of health. Macmillan, Basingstoke

Gough P 1994 Class and social policy. In: Gough P, Maslin-Prothero S, Masterton A (eds) Nursing and social policy: care in context. Butterworth Heinemann, London

Graham H 1993 Hardship and health in women's lives. Harvester Wheatsheaf, Brighton

Grimsley M, Bhatt A 1988 Health. In: Bhatt A, Carr-Hill R, Ohri S (eds) Britain's black population. Gower, Aldershot

Ham C 1992 Health policy in Britain; the politics and organisation of the National Health Service. Macmillan, Basingstoke

LeGrande J 1982 The strategy of equality: redistribution and the social services. Allen & Unwin, London

McNaught A 1987 Health action and ethnic minorities. Bedford Square Press, London

Mann M 1987 Ruling class strategies and citizenship. Sociology 21(3): 339–354

Marshall T 1950 Citizenship and social class. Cambridge University Press, Cambridge

Maslin-Prothero S 1994 Race and policy. In: Gough P, Maslin-Prothero S, Masterson A (eds) Nursing and social policy, care in context. Butterworth, Heinmann, London

Mishra R 1977 Society and social policy: theories and practice of welfare. Macmillan, London

Neave J 1994 Older people. In: Gough P, Maslin-Prothero S, Masterson A (eds) Nursing and social policy: Care in context. Butterworth, Heinmann, London

Nettleton S 1995 The sociology of health and illness. Polity Press, Cambridge

Oliver M 1990 The politics of disablement. Macmillan, Basingstoke

OPCS 1986 Occupational mortality: dicennial supplement 1979–80, 1982–83. HMSO, London

OPCS 1988 Occupational mortality: childhood supplement 1979–80, 1982–83. HMSO, London

Parker G 1992 With due care and attention. SPRU, York

Pascall G 1986 Social policy: a feminist analysis. Tavistock, London

Pearson M 1986 The politics of ethnic minority health studies. In: Rathwell T, Phillips D (eds) Health, race and ethnicity. Croom Helm, London

Popay J, Jones G 1990 Patterns of wealth and illness among lone parents. Journal of Social Policy 19: 499–534

Smart D 1987 Sickle-cell anaemia – women speak out. In: O'Sullivan S (ed) Women's health: a spare rib reader. Pandora Press, London

Taylor D 1989 Citizenship and social power. Critical Social Policy 9: 19–31

Taylor-Gooby 1991 Social change, social welfare and social science. Harvester Wheatsheaf, London

Thomas-Hope E 1992 International migration and health: sickle-cell and thalassemia health care in the UK. Geo Journal 26(1): 75–79

Torkington P 1987 Blaming black women: rickets and racism. In: O'Sullivan S (ed) Women's health: a spare rib reader. Pandora Press, London

Townsend P, Davidson N 1992 The Black report. In: Inequalities in Health. Penguin, London

Turner B 1990 Outline of a theory of citizenship. Sociology 24(2):189–217

Walby S 1990 Theorising Patriarchy. Blackwell, Oxford

Walby S 1994 Is citizenship gendered? Sociology 28(2): 379–395

Walker A 1987 A social construction of dependency in old age. In: Loney M (ed) The state or the market? Politics of welfare in contemporary Britain. Sage, London

Walker A 1993 Community care policy: from consensus to conflict. In: Bornat B, Pereira C, Pilgrim D, Williams F (eds) Community care: a reader. Macmillan, Basingstoke

White A, Nicolaas G, Foster K, Cary S 1993 Health survey for England 1991. HMSO, London

Whitehead M 1987 The health divide. In: Inequalities in Health. Penguin, London

Wicks M 1987 Family matters and public policy. In: Loney M (ed) The state of the market? Politics and welfare in contemporary Britain. Sage, London

Williams F 1989 Social policy: a critical introduction. Polity Press, Cambridge

Williams F 1992 Somewhere over the rainbow. In: Manning N, Page R (eds) Social Policy Review 4. Longman, London

7 The Social Interpretation of Deviance

Sam Porter

Key concepts

- Theories of symbolic interactionism
- Theories of labelling and the social processes of mental illness
- Deviance and disability
- Total institutions
- Control and care

One way of classifying sociological approaches is to distinguish between those that concentrate on social determination and those that emphasise social interpretation. Examination of social determination involves looking at how society causes various things to happen in our lives. This was the approach taken in Chapter 5, where it was shown how aspects of society such as poverty and inequality caused ill-health in those who were disadvantaged. By contrast, this chapter concentrates on the social interpretation of ill-health. Social interpretivism involves the belief that the world as we experience it is not something out there that everybody can interpret in the same way. The way that we interpret what is going on around us (and indeed within us) will be affected by the way that we have been brought up and educated. In short, the type of society that we live in will have a great deal of influence over the way that we interpret our world. One of the ways of demonstrating that this is the case is to show how members of societies interpret different things and behaviours in radically different ways. Take sex, for example. You might think that it is just a matter of biological drives, but as Berger & Luckmann (1971) note, it is far more than that:

'While man [sic] possesses sexual drives that are comparable to those of the other higher mammals, human sexuality is characterised by a very high

degree of pliability ... [The] evidence shows that, in sexual matters, man is capable of almost anything. One may stimulate one's sexual imagination to a pitch of feverish lust, but it is unlikely that one can conjure up any image that will not correspond to what in some other culture is an established norm, or at least an occurrence to be taken in its stride. At the same time, of course, human sexuality is directed, sometimes rigidly structured, in every particular culture. Every culture has a distinctive sexual configuration, with its own specialised pattern of sexual conduct ... The empirical relativity of these configurations, their immense variety and luxurious inventiveness, indicate that they are a product of man's own socio-cultural formations rather than of a biologically fixed human nature.'
(Berger & Luckmann 1971:67)

This approach can also be applied to illness and abnormal behaviour. As nurses, we are no more immune to social interpretations of reality than other members of society. However, as nurses, we also have a responsibility to question our interpretations of people who are or who behave in ways that are interpreted as being the result of illness. The primary aim of this chapter is to try to uncover some of the assumptions that are made about various groups of people who require nursing care. However, before doing this, it is necessary to examine in a little more detail the theoretical ideas that underpin this approach to the social interpretation of illness.

Symbolic Interactionism

It will be remembered from Chapter 4 that one of the main strands of social interpretivism was that of **symbolic interactionism**. Symbolic interactionists have made a considerable contribution to our understanding of how the sick and the 'deviant' are interpreted by other members of society, and, as a result, their findings will loom large in this chapter. In order to understand where these sociologists are coming from, it is necessary to have a grasp of the fundamentals of symbolic interactionism as a social theory.

The Symbolic Interactionism of Herbert Blumer

The term 'symbolic interactionism' was first coined by the American sociologist Herbert Blumer. Blumer argued that what is unique about human beings is their capacity to think about and consider what is going on around them. This unique capacity comes about because humans have the capacity to create and manipulate symbols. Symbols are abstract representations of outside reality which are shared among groups of people.

The most important symbols are those of language. Because of their capacity to use and understand symbols, when people respond to the actions of others, they do not do so in an automatic fashion. Rather, their response is based on the meaning that the action has for them 'Thus, human interaction is mediated by the use of symbols, by interpretation, or by ascertaining the meaning of one another's actions' (Blumer 1962:180). Hence the name 'symbolic interactionism'.

This might all sound a bit complicated and philosophical. Perhaps the best way to understand what symbolic interactionism is all about is to go through the three basic premises of this social theory, as laid out by Blumer (1969). The first premise was that 'human beings act towards things on the basis of the meanings that the things have for them' (1969:2). By 'things' he did not just mean physical objects, but also other human beings, ideas, activities and situations. Basically, all Blumer is saying here is that we use our minds when we act. Rather than reacting in a reflex fashion, we interpret what is going on around us and act on the basis of the interpretation that we make. This might seem a fairly obvious point. However, Blumer argued that it was a point that many sociology scholars had forgotten, which led them to tend to see people's behaviour as determined solely by outside factors, such as social structures. Blumer rejected this position, arguing that rather than being the puppets of external forces, human beings are active in their own right. He argued that, in order to understand behaviour, we need to do more than simply identify the outside factors that influence that behaviour. Because the meanings that things have for people are crucial in their own right, an adequate explanation of behaviour must take account of them.

It can be seen that the first premise of symbolic interactionism placed great importance on the meanings that people attached to things. The next obvious question is: where do these meanings come from? The second premise of symbolic interactionism involved a rejection of the idea that meaning came from the intrinsic qualities of things; that, for example, the meaning that the human body has for us is the sole result of the body's anatomy and physiology of which we can have direct and accurate understanding. Blumer also rejected the idea that meaning was generated solely by the minds of individual people; that, for example, each one of us simply makes up our own understanding of the body, depending on how our individual mind decides to interpret it. Instead, he argued that meaning arises from the process of interaction between people. From the day they are born, people gain their understanding of the world around them by taking on board the attitudes and responses of others. Our understanding of the world is not natural in the sense that the symbols that we use to understand the world are human rather than natural constructs. Thus, Blumer sees meanings as social products, as creations that are formed in and through defining activities of people as they interact (Blumer 1969:4–5).

The second premise gives the social world in which people live a great deal of significance; because the meanings on which we base our actions are social products, our social environment is central to the way we understand the world. Such a premise might seem to stand in contradiction to the first premise, the main thrust of which was to reject the assumption that humans automatically adopt the ideas that are current in the society they live in, and are incapable of thinking for themselves, where the meanings that things have for people are socially determined.

The third premise, that 'meanings are handled in, and modified through, an interpretative process used by the person in dealing with the things he [sic] encounters' (1969:2), seeks to resolve the tension between the first and second premises. According to Blumer, the ideas that we get from our interaction with other members of our society do not determine the way that we act; rather, they are better seen as instruments that guide our actions. He argues that the 'interpretative process' involves what might be termed an internal conversation in which the person interacts with her/himself, and thinks about her/his own attitudes and understandings. One of the defining characteristics of human beings is the capacity to reflect on one's own mental processes. On the basis of this internal communication, the person is able to select, modify, check or reject socially generated meanings in the light of her/his situation and aims. This means that there is nothing automatic about our use of meanings – rather than accepting them without question, we revise and adapt them.

Reflection point 7.1

The three premises of symbolic interactionism:

1. We usually act on the basis of our interpretation of a situation, rather than on the basis of an unthinking reflex response.
2. We learn to interpret the world through our interaction with those around us.
3. Because we are able to reflect on our interpretations, they may be different from those of the people around us.

Labelling Theory

On the basis of the general theoretical foundations of symbolic interactionism as formulated by Blumer, we can now move on to examine how this approach can be used by nurses to understand their own interactions with clients. The first area that is discussed involves the application of what has been termed **labelling** theory, and how this can be applied in order to illuminate the social processes that lie behind someone being diagnosed and treated as mentally ill. However, before discussing the specific example of mental illness, we need to address the more general issue of deviance. This is useful both because the labelling theory of deviance provides the basis for much symbolic interactionist work on mental illness, but also because it can, in itself, be usefully applied to other health issues pertinent to nursing such as illegal drug use and sexual deviance.

One of the most important sociologists in the development of labelling theory was the American sociologist Howard Becker (in contrast to many other sociological positions, which have a European origin, symbolic interactionism is a home-grown American product). Becker built his labelling theory of deviance from two basic symbolic interactionist premises.

1. How we see the world and act within it is the result of neither biology nor external social forces, but rather of the interpretations that emerge from our interaction with others.
2. The meaning that we attach to a person or a thing is not the result of the internal qualities of that person or thing, but of the active interpretations that we put upon them.

Accordingly, he regarded deviance from social norms not as a given fact but as a result of the interpretations that members of society apply to certain individuals. The following reflection point is derived from Becker's work.

Reflection point 7.2	'Deviance is *not* a quality of the act the person commits, but rather a consequence of the application by others of rules and sanctions to an "offender". The deviant is one to whom that label has been successfully applied; deviant behaviour is behaviour that people so label.' (Becker 1963:9)

It should be stressed that Becker was not implying that people labelled as deviant had not committed the act that they were accused of committing. However, he was arguing that we could not assume that this was the case. Because the process of labelling is not infallible, people might be labelled without having broken the social rule that they have been accused of breaking. Similarly, people may break rules and get away with it, thus avoiding the label being applied to them. If we accept this argument, the interesting question no longer concerns the factors that can account for a supposed act of deviance. Rather, such an analysis concentrates on 'deviance as the product of a transaction that takes place between some social group and one who is viewed by the group as a rule-breaker' (Becker 1963:10).

Becker believes that whether an act is deviant or not has little to do with the act itself. Instead, it depends on how other people react to the act. This approach to deviance is not the way that most of us think about it. We tend to explain deviance in terms of the actions of the people that we regard as being deviant. Thus, for example, it might seem cut and dried to us that someone who regularly uses heroin is deviant because of the fact that they use it, not because other members of society tend to interpret heroin use as deviant. Yet, if we think about it, there are surely many heroin users (not least among those who can gain easy access to it, namely health-care workers) who carry on their lives without ever being regarded as deviant – the deviants are only those users that we get to know about.

Once people are uncovered and exposed as deviants, this often has profound consequences for their lives. This issue has been addressed by Edwin Lemert (1967), who distinguishes between what he calls *primary deviance* and *secondary deviance*. Lemert argues that lots of us break social rules, but this does not make us deviants. Our inflections are overlooked, excused in various ways, or simply not attended to. However, sometimes, a person's rule-breaking is attended to and becomes a major factor in how people subsequently deal with them. For example, someone may be a husband, father, golf-player, consultant oncologist and general pillar of society, and also someone who takes some recreational heroin from time to time. At this stage his drug use only involves primary deviance, in that it has little or no effect on his other social roles. But if he is caught, his other roles may be forgotten and subordinated to the role of drug abuser. If charged and convicted of illegal drug use, he may have his name struck from the medical register, thus losing his livelihood. He may be blackballed from the golf club, and his wife may leave him and his children reject him. Now his drug use is a major part of what he is – he is in a state of secondary deviation. He has moved from somebody who occasionally does deviant things to being a deviant. Lemert's central point is that there is a difference between committing deviant acts and being a deviant. The key from moving from primary to secondary deviation is labelling.

According to Lemert, labelling not only defines deviance, but may cause further deviation. Returning to symbolic interactionist theory, this

Reflection point 7.3	Bring to mind recent (and not so recent) instances where well-known and/or well-respected people have been labelled as deviant through drug misuse, promiscuity, or forms of sexual behaviour that fall outside society's expected norms. Do you feel that society expects different standards of behaviour from certain groups such as pop stars, politicians, or priests and as such attaches the deviant label selectively?

involves the assumption that people have a tendency to see themselves in a way that others see them. Our sense of who we are is a social product, in that we construct the world by taking on board the images that others in the world offer us. Thus, if you treat a child as if he (or she) were stupid for long enough, he tends to become stupid because he internalises that image of himself. Someone who is labelled as deviant and treated accordingly may come to see himself as that sort of person and therefore become more fixed in his deviant ways. This is especially likely to happen when rejection by conventional society is accompanied by being welcomed into a deviant subculture. One obvious reason for getting involved in a deviant subculture is that it provides the resources for one's deviance. If you are a drug-taker, then you want to be involved in a drug subculture because you need to obtain your drugs. However, there is a more subtle sociopsychological reason for being drawn to a deviant subculture, in that, ironically, it is the very place where a person's deviant status ceases to be the main focus of attention. Take people with a physical disability, for example. Even in settings where their disability should make no difference, they are still regarded as different by others, who see their disability as the most significant thing about them. How can disabled people get away from this irritating obsession with their 'deviant' status? The best way of doing so is to associate with people of a similar status. Other disabled people do not categorise you solely in terms of your disability, but are prepared to interact with you on the basis of all your other characteristics.

Reflection point 7.4

The medical model of disability seems to regard the person with disability as somehow 'tragic'. Christopher Goodall (1995) describes well-worn phrases such as 'crippled with arthritis' as being representative of this 'tragedy' model. He goes on to say how much the media love 'heroic cripples' who fight against disablement to beat the odds stacked against them. He writes of one newspaper greeting his wheelchair ascent of a Pennine hill as 'Crippled Chris Conquers Wild Boar Fell'.

Do you feel that misplaced sentiments of this kind serve only to exacerbate the labelling process?

There are lessons for nurses to be learnt from these observations. How do we and how should we treat our patients? Is it valid to reduce people to the status of 'the parasuicide', or 'the Down syndrome in bed 5'? Often the cause for a person coming into contact with nurses is also seen by many members of society as involving a deviant attribute. Often nurses reinforce the labelling of deviance by concentrating solely on that attribute in their interactions with patients. One of the benefits of holistic

**Activity
7.1**

Question 1: In general, do you think it is important for health-care staff to be aware of the drugs that their patients are taking? Give reasons for your answer.

Imagine that you are a regular non-intravenous user of heroin who has just been admitted to hospital suffering from an acute asthmatic attack. While your knowledge of asthma is not too great, you do not think there is a direct connection between heroin use and asthma, although you believe that too much heroin can slow down your breathing. You work for an insurance company, and you are worried about them finding out about your secret habit.

Question 2: Would you tell your admitting nurse about your drug use?

Give reasons for your decision.

Did your answers to questions 1 and 2 match up?

If not, why not, and what could be done to make them match?

care, which seeks to widen nursing attention away from the specifics of disease, is that it enables nurses to see the other aspects that make up the people they care for, and therefore tends to minimise rather than reinforce the effects of deviant status.

One problem with Lemert's view of deviance is that it appears rather deterministic. It would seem that, once the label of deviance has been applied, the person so labelled is on the rocky road to ruin and there is little that he or she can do about it. In other words, once a label has been applied, it becomes fixed. This is the sort of approach taken by Felicity Stockwell in her classic study, 'The Unpopular Patient' (Stockwell 1972), which demonstrated the degree to which nurses apply labels to their patients, which often have damaging consequences for their care. Stockwell's research, carried out on general wards, sought to uncover the traits displayed by patients that were likely to lead to them being labelled as 'good' (popular patients) or 'bad' (unpopular patients).

Among the most significant traits she identified were being of foreign nationality, having been in hospital for more than three months, and having a psychiatric diagnosis. For Stockwell the issue was rather clear-cut: 'It is possible to identify patients who are popular and unpopular with the nurses' (Stockwell 1972:30). However, in a recent reconsideration of the issue of the unpopular patient, Johnson & Webb (1995) discovered that the process of labelling patients good or bad was considerably more fluid than might be expected from examination of Stockwell's work:

> 'Labels are pluralistic. By this we mean that patients were capable of being evaluated on more than one level even by the same individual. Physically they could be unpopular because of the difficulties involved in performing their care, but interpersonally they were liked, perhaps because they were stoical or humorous. Labels were uncertain in another sense, that there was no true consensus over the evaluations. Frequently nurses would suggest that privately they really liked someone who had been defined elsewhere as "unpopular"'.
> (Johnson & Webb 1995:472)

This observation is not to say that there was no pattern to the process at all. Johnson and Webb observed that some nurses had more power than others to ensure that their evaluation of a patient carried weight. The notion of power and the process of decision making is discussed later in the book.

Mental Illness as Labelled Deviance

One of the more controversial areas to which labelling theory has been applied has been that of mental illness. Labelling theorists such as Thomas Scheff do not see the symptoms of mental illness as results of psychological problems, but as 'labelled violations of social norms' (Scheff 1966:25). Scheff called the type of social norms involved 'residual rules'. These are the most basic of social conventions, which are considered so 'natural' that they are not governed by explicit rules. For example, Scheff argues that one of the basic conventions in life is that when one is in a public place, one should at least appear to have a purpose to one's activities. Thus, there is a residual rule against having no purpose. Of course, this rule is not explicit – it is not written down on any legal statute. Nevertheless, people go to great lengths to adhere to it. Even when people are in effect loafing around doing nothing, they usually adopt strategies that will put a respectable veneer on their lack of purpose. Instead of sitting by a river bank, people fish; instead of sleeping on a beach, they 'get a tan'. By contrast, those who hang about in public without an acceptable pretext for doing so are seen as violating a residual rule. According to Scheff because they violate this rule, their actions may be interpreted as symptoms of mental illness. This will bring them to the attention of the psychiatric authorities.

You might argue that it is reasonable to use odd behaviour in public places as a possible indicator of mental health problems, and that there is nothing wrong in investigating whether or not this is the case. Scheff's retort to this is that there is little justification in singling such people out. This is because we all, at some time or another, break residual rules.

However, we are not all labelled as mentally ill. There must therefore be something more to the diagnosis of mental illness than the actions that are used as a justification for that diagnosis.

Scheff argues that the most important single factor that leads some residual rule-breakers to be labelled as deviant lies not in the behaviour of the rule-breaker, but in the reaction of other members of society. This reaction involves the application of the stereotype of mental illness. Whether or not this stereotype is applied depends on a number of factors, including the amount of tolerance that the community has for the act committed, the status and power of the rule-breaker, and the availability of alternative explanations. Once labelled as mentally ill Scheff argues that the person has been launched on a deviant 'career'. Those who are labelled will usually be rewarded for adopting the stereotypical role of mental illness, whereas, if they attempt to resist it and assert their normality, they will tend to be punished.

Scheff's labelling theory of mental illness has not been accepted by all sociologists. For example, Walter Gove (1980) has argued that Scheff's description of the career of the mental patient is simply incorrect. Gove is not persuaded that mental illness can be explained solely in terms of residual rule-breaking, noting that the majority of people so labelled quite evidently have a serious disorder, which frequently causes them a great deal of unhappiness. In addition, he argues that instead of being coerced into adopting the stereotype of mental illness, many people are

Reflection point 7.5

In a study to examine the accuracy of psychiatric diagnosis, eight people behaved in such a way that they were admitted to twelve different mental hospitals in the United States. They did this by ringing the hospitals up and complaining that they had been hearing voices. However, after being admitted, these 'pseudopatients' acted normally and made no more complaints about hearing voices. Despite this, in all but one case, they were diagnosed as being schizophrenic. They were kept in hospital for an average of two and a half weeks; during this time the fact that they were behaving normally was never detected by those caring for them. When they were discharged, rather than being given a clean bill of health, they were labelled as having 'schizophrenia in remission'. When the staff of one hospital discovered what had happened, they claimed that the experiment was unfair, and that if they had realised that pseudopatients were going to be admitted they would have been able to detect them. They were told that in the next three months at least one pseudopatient would attempt to get himself or herself admitted. During this period, over 10% of admissions were labelled as pseudopatients by a least one psychiatrist. Yet in that period no pseudopatients attempted to gain admission. (Rosenhan 1973) screened out by mental health professionals and many others, following treatment, are able to put their experiences behind them, without becoming institutionalised.

Total Institutions

Another symbolic interactionist interpretation of the experience of mental illness has been given by Erving Goffman in his famous book, 'Asylums' (1968a). In examining what he terms the moral career of the mental patient, Goffman concentrates on 'the regular sequence of changes that career entails in the person's self and in his framework of imagery for judging himself and others' (1968a:119). Like Scheff, Goffman uses the term 'career' not in the sense of occupational development, but rather in the more general sense of referring to any strand of a person's course through life. Goffman identifies three major stages in this moral career: pre-patient, in-patient and ex-patient. Concentrating on the first two stages, Goffman graphically demonstrates the 'mortification of the self' – the stripping away of a person's original identity – that is involved. In the pre-patient stage, a typical scenario would be close relatives or friends coming to the decision that the pre-patient's behaviour or beliefs indicate that psychiatric care is appropriate. This has a dramatic effect on the pre-patient's interpersonal relationships and sense of self. As Goffman puts it:

> 'he [sic] starts out with relationships and rights, and ends up, at the beginning of his hospital stay, with hardly any of either. The moral aspects of this career, then, typically begin with the experience of abandonment, disloyalty and embitterment.'
> (Goffman 1968a:125)

What is hardest to bear is what pre-patients often see as the betrayal of those closest to them. They discover that those who they rely on for help when they are threatened with institutionalisation, are themselves often involved in the admission process, in collaboration with psychiatric professionals. Thus, the comforts and certainties of the pre-patient's world are stripped away, to the point where the pre-patient may conclude 'that he has been deserted by society and turned out of relationships by those closest to him' (Goffman 1968a:135).

This process of the 'mortification of the self' continues during the in-patient stage. This stage involves the person entering what Goffman calls a **total institution** – an institution cut off from the rest of the social world, where inmates work, rest and play in the same place, surrounded by a large number of fellow inmates who are all treated alike, and where the daily activities of life are tightly governed by formal rules which are enforced by the institution's officials.

One of the consequences of entering such an institution is that the usual props of personality, such as freedom of movement, personalised clothing and privacy are denied. In-patients begin to realise how difficult it is to see themselves as human individuals when the usual social supports for individuality are removed. Moreover, it is impressed on them that they are failures, and therefore no longer deserving of the status normally accorded to adult members of society. In reaction to this, patients may try to construct a version of their past which minimises their personal responsibility for what has happened to them with the aim of reducing the shame they are experiencing. However, according to Goffman, these attempts by in-patients to present themselves as respectable human beings conflict with the interests of professional staff, who want patients to accept their weaknesses as they have been defined by staff and as a result to cooperate with the psychiatric treatments that have been prescribed to cure those weaknesses. Because of this, staff have much to gain from undermining patients' attempts to maintain respectable images of themselves. They do this by challenging claims which involve the denial of responsibility, and by emphasising those aspects of a person's history that are most discrediting.

In general then, mental hospitals systematically provide for circulation about each patient the kind of information that the patient is likely to try to hide. And in various degrees of detail this information is used daily to puncture his (or her) claims. At the admission and diagnostic conferences, he will be asked questions to which he must give wrong answers in order to maintain his self-respect, and then the true answer will be shot back at him (Goffman 1968a:148).

If patients attempt to reconstruct their story of respectability after this sort of assault upon it, the process may well be repeated again, with their new story being discredited by staff. Goffman identifies two possible outcomes of this process. One is a situation in which patients accept that the only chance they have of regaining a creditable self-image is to fully accept the views of the professionals that are looking after them. In this scenario, the self is reborn as a model patient.

The other possible outcome is one where, in Goffman's words, patients learn to practise 'the amoral arts of shamelessness' (1968a:155). Here, patients come to the realisation that they can survive without what they would previously have seen as essential, namely self-respect. As a consequence, they give up serious attempts at defending themselves against the efforts of psychiatric staff to debunk that self-respect. From this perspective of apathy, the process of building up a self just to have it destroyed simply becomes a shameless game.

We should be wary of assuming that 'Asylum' provides us with an accurate description of *contemporary* psychiatric health care. After all it was written over 35 years ago and the nature of care has changed considerably since then. Indeed, it should be noted that 'Asylum' itself has made a considerable contribution to the changing of attitudes towards psychiatric institutions over the last three decades. During this period, there has been an increasing emphasis on the benefits of community care, which, it might be argued, has altered the dynamics of professional/client interaction. Consider, for example, the Case study 7.1.

Case study 7.1	Fifty-one-year-old James was diagnosed as having schizophrenia when he was in his early twenties. Initially, he experienced several lengthy periods of in-patient care within a traditional mental hospital where electroconvulsive therapy and major tranquillisers were the treatment of choice. During this early part of his illness the label 'schizophrenic' became firmly attached and this has stayed with him to the present day. When he was not in hospital James lived with his parents. Because of negative, often hurtful reactions to him by neighbours James became a recluse, only going out during the periods of darkness for short walks. Eventually, his ordinary everyday behaviours were re-interpreted by neighbours who voiced their concerns about his deterioration to his parents. The neighbours were also heard to complain about his nightime wanderings and to say that they were afraid of his intentions.

Points to consider:
This case study provides an example of the reality of the concepts primary and secondary deviance. Nurses working in the field of mental health need to consider the impact of negative labelling on the quality of life for individual clients and take into consideration the possibility of a 'courtesy stigma' ascribed to families of stigmatised individuals.

However, it would be a mistake to assume that institutions no longer pose problems for the individuals that live in them. It is not just the mentally ill who have been subjected to the process of de-personalisation. Another vulnerable group who have much contact with nurses are the elderly. This issue has been addressed by Alistair Hewison (1995) in a study of nurse–patient interactions. In this paper, Hewison seeks to uncover the manifestations of power in professional/client encounters. He approaches this issue from the symbolic interactionist perspective that the social world is a process of varied interactions, rather than a fixed structure, arguing that 'social reality is created through interaction and is constantly being negotiated and defined' (Hewison 1995:76).

After observing interactions between nurses and older women on a 'care of the elderly' ward, Hewison identified four different interactional strategies that nurses adopted in order to exercise power over their clients. The first strategy, which he terms 'overt power', involved nurses openly giving orders or making decisions without consulting patients. In the latter strategy, nursing power is the result of 'an expectation on the part of the nurse, and an acceptance on the part of the patient, that the nurse will be in control' (Hewison 1995:78). Thus, we can see that overt power is not simply a matter of making people do things against their will. In many cases, patients interpreted nurses' open power as legitimate, and willingly went along with it.

Hewison terms the second strategy used by nurses 'persuasion'. This involves nurses cajoling patients to do things that they originally did not want to do. Of course, there is nothing unusual or necessarily sinister about interactions between people involving negotiations and attempts at persuasion. However, we once again need to look at the balance of power within the relationship. Hewison argues that nurses' position within the organisation of health care gives them a pegged position in the negotiating process.

The third strategy involves 'controlling the agenda'. Hewison argues that this is the most common way that nurses exert power over elderly patients. In this case the exercise of power is very subtle and comes in the form of manipulation. Controlling the agenda involves appearing to give patients a choice by asking questions, but constructing the questions in such a way that, in reality, patients have little choice but to go along with what nurses want them to do.

The final strategy, 'terms of endearment', is probably the most subtle of all, in that it is often based on displays of affection. This strategy involves nurses interpreting their relationship with patients as being similar to that of the relationship between parents and children. If such an interpretation is accepted by patients, then nurses' control is further legitimated in the eyes of both – control and care become two sides of the one coin.

How should we view this rather depressing account of the care of older people? Certainly, Hewison's study gives us a clear insight into the ways that nurses interpret their relationship with older patients, and how they attempt to manipulate the understandings of elderly patients so as to ensure that their behaviour fits with what the nurses feel is appropriate. However, the study gives us little insight into how the elderly women observed actively interpreted the world. Just as in Goffman's work, the interaction seems to be a matter of one-way traffic. Hewison is aware of this problem:

'The data presented . . . may seem to suggest that the exercise of power was totally one way. This was not the case and sometimes patients did exert control, but this was a rare occurrence.'
(Hewison 1995:80)

The fact that nurses' power was usually successfully applied, and that patients' perspectives had little influence on subsequent action, might lead us to question whether or not symbolic interactionism can take sufficient account of the significance of coercion in social life. In contrast to Blumer's position that people are not passive recipients of external determining factors, but active creators of their own reality, both these studies seem to show just how much influence external factors can have on people's behaviour in certain circumstances, irrespective of how they themselves wish to interpret the situation.

| **Activity 7.2** | 'Total institutions disrupt and defile precisely those actions that in civil society have the role of attesting to the actor and those in his presence that he has some command over his world – that he is a person with "adult" self-determination, autonomy and freedom of action.' (Goffman 1968a:47) |

Imagine that you have just been appointed Ward Manager of a long-stay care of the elderly unit. What would you do to ensure that your patients' images of themselves as autonomous adults is neither disrupted nor defiled? Some areas you might care to think about are:
- Clothing
- Personal hygiene
- Eating
- Sleeping
- Mobility
- Outside contact
- Interaction

Stigma

We saw from Goffman's account of the mortification of the self that takes place in total institutions that one of the most important aspects of people's humanity is their self-respect. Goffman returned to this theme in his extremely influential book dealing with the issue of social **stigma**. In 'Stigma' (Goffman 1968b), Goffman examines the effects on an individual that result from the application to him or her of a stigmatising label which challenges his or her self-respect.

At the centre of Goffman's model of the human self was his belief first that our sense of ourselves is closely bound up with how others see us and, second, that we realise this is so. In order to foster a sense of self-esteem we will therefore make an effort to present ourselves to others as worthy of esteem. Goffman calls this strategy of presenting ourselves in the best light 'impression management' (1968b). It involves performing in such a way as to control the impression that others have of us that will lead them to approve of us. It should be noted that this view of the self has radical implications – rather than seeing people's personalities as authentic and relatively stable, Goffman sees the human self as a series of roles or parts, which will change depending on our audience. In short, life is just a series of dramatic performances. For example, the person confronted in a hospital emergency admission bed will be playing the role of 'patient'. In doing so, that person may be radically different in terms of her (or his) personality and behaviour compared to what she was a few hours ago when she was playing the role of, for example, 'managing director' at work which in turn was almost completely different from the role they were playing that morning as 'loving wife and mother'. For most of us for most of the time, our impression management works. However, for many people, impression management is not so easy. These are people who have been stigmatised.

What does Goffman mean when he talks about stigma? Goffman argues that in every society there exist commonly held stereotypes, or simplistic generalisations. These stereotypes include expectations about how individuals ought to be. However, some people's social identities do not match the stereotypical expectations of the society they live in. It is this gap between social expectations and the attributes a person has that generates stigma. This is not simply a matter of difference; it also implies a moral judgement in that stigma is a difference that is deeply discrediting. Indeed, Goffman goes so far as to argue that we do not see people with stigmas as fully human. The view that the stigmatised are inferior to what he terms 'normals' results in all sorts of discrimination, and rationalisations for that discrimination. Nor is it just 'normals' who accept this moral evaluation. The stigmatised themselves are unable to escape the stereotypes of the society they live in, so they tend to see themselves as inferior and shameful.

Just as Becker did not see deviance as the result of a specific act, but as a result of the social response to that act, so Goffman does not see stigma as the result of a specific attribute that a person possesses, but the result of the social interpretation of that attribute. Thus, for example, many people would find the need for psychiatric care, which usually brings with it the label of mental illness, a very stigmatising experience. However, if one is a well-heeled New Yorker, attending a psychoanalyst is not met with this sort of disapproval; indeed, it is almost a status symbol. This is because the stereotypes that exist in middle class New York society lead people to look upon what is essentially the same act in a completely different way.

Stigma is not an issue to be taken lightly. It deeply affects the lives of those who have been stigmatised. For them, dealing with 'normals' is often highly difficult and uncomfortable. One of the difficulties is that the stigma will be in the forefront of both their minds. This has at least two effects. First, it makes the stigmatised feel very self-conscious. Second, it can distort the normal's interpretation of what should be everyday events, whereby a minor accomplishment by the stigmatised is seen as an amazing achievement, whereas a minor failing is interpreted as a direct result of the person's stigmatised difference. Paradoxically, it is likely that at the same time the normal will pretend not even to notice the discredited attribute of the stigmatised. This very self-conscious 'disattention' adds to the difficulties of interaction, causing tensions, uncertainties and ambiguities for those involved, and especially for the stigmatised person. It can be seen that impression management of what Goffman terms a 'spoiled identity' is full of difficulties and hazards. Often the anticipation of difficulties is so great that the stigmatised actively avoids contact with others. This results in even more problems, such as depression and anxiety, that are the result of social isolation.

Activity 7.3

You are caring for a group of patients with a nursing colleague who suffers from eczema. One of these patients, a middle-aged man, informs you that, because of her skin complaint, he does not wish to be washed by your colleague.

What should you say to the patient?

What should you say to your colleague?

Fortunately there are people with whom the stigmatised can interact without encountering these difficulties. These are people who see the stigmatised not as discredited but as 'properly human'. Goffman divides these people into two categories – the 'own' and the 'wise'. The own are those who are similarly stigmatised, and who therefore know what it feels like from first hand experience. The wise are those who are 'normal' but whose particular situation gives them access to, and sympathy for, the hidden life of the stigmatised individual and who come to accept them for what they are. One group of wise people are those who work in an occupation that caters for the wants of the stigmatised. It is into this category that nurses may fit. Of course, the development from familiarity to acceptance is not an automatic process.

Not all attributes open to social stigma are immediately apparent. Those people whose differentness is not immediately apparent are termed by Goffman as being 'discreditable' (in contrast to those whose difference is evident – the 'discredited'). For the discreditable, impression management involves working out just how much information about themselves it is wise or safe to disclose to others. One approach to this situation is what Goffman calls 'passing' (as normal), and pretending to others that they do not have the attribute that they regard as stigmatising.

Examples of this might be of the person who is hard of hearing who wears a hearing aid, or the person with diabetes who administers his or her insulin injections secretly. Often, passing strategies will be developed in collaboration with close relatives or friends who are 'in the know'. For example, the partner of a person with a colostomy may routinely check for odours before the person leaves the house. However, there is always the danger that the stigma will become publicly known in spite of the person's best efforts. For example, a person with diabetes mellitus who suffers a public hypoglycaemic attack will pass dramatically and embarrassingly from discreditable to discredited.

Rather than constantly living in fear of exposure, some people prefer to manage disclosure of information on their own terms, which means that they can simultaneously attempt to minimise the obtrusiveness of the stigma. Goffman terms this strategy covering. He uses the example of a facially disfigured blind person who chooses to wear dark glasses in public. The glasses in this case serve the dual purpose of indicating the person's blindness, but also hiding his disfigurement.

Schneider & Conrad (1981) have expanded on Goffman's model of discreditable with reference to people with epilepsy. They supplement Goffman's model with the distinction between 'adjusted' and 'unadjusted' adaptation of individuals to their illness. They argue that both passing and covering (or 'secret' and 'pragmatic' adaptation in their terms) are types of more or less successful adjustment. To these they add the category of 'quasi-liberated', in which people make no attempt to hide their epilepsy, but instead reject the stigma, challenging the ideas of others and attempting to educate them. However, in contrast to these three modes of adjustment, which all involve a definite strategy for coping with the stigma of epilepsy, Schneider and Conrad noted that some individuals are simply overwhelmed by the consequences of their illness. These fell into the category of unadjusted adaptation. Epilepsy takes over their lives, and has a severely negative impact on them. Schneider and Conrad observe that this 'debilitated response' is very similar to Lemert's secondary deviation:

> 'in that the debilitated response embraces epilepsy as an indelible and irrevocable threat to one's worth; it pursues epilepsy as a deviant, stigmatising and debilitating blemish or flaw, as a 'cross to bear.'
> (Schneider & Conrad 1981:217)

Another example of the unfortunate effects of stigma can be found In Edgerton's (1967) examination of the lives of mentally handicapped people. Edgerton noted that the mentally handicapped were well aware that they were the subject of social stigma. As a result they made brave attempts to reduce this stigma by passing themselves of as 'normal'.

Unfortunately, for the most part, these efforts were unsuccessful. However, their fragile attempts to create the image of normality were bolstered by sympathetic people around them who engaged in a 'benevolent conspiracy' in which it was pretended that efforts to display normality were more successful than they actually were.

Summary

We can see from Goffman's work on stigma that symbolic interactionist insights into the degree to which our individual selves are bound up with those around us leads to distressing problems when those around us fail to afford us full recognition of our humanity. This approach to the social interpretation of deviance alerts us as nurses to our responsibilities. If our duty is to enable those in our care to cope with the problems which beset them then we have a responsibility to be aware of the importance of labelling and stigma to the experience of illness, and to do what we can to reduce their consequences upon the lives of individuals.

Of course, the interpretative approach may sometimes be pushed too far by those who advocate it. Certainly, some commentators such as Erving Zeitlin (1973) and Anthony Giddens (1984) have argued that Goffman's view of life as perpetual play-acting underestimates the coherence of the human character – that there is more to us than the act that we are happening to put on at any one time. Nevertheless, given that the attitudes of others are so important to sufferers' experience of illness or disability, the moral of the story is that nurses should think very carefully about their own attitudes and the manner in which they portray them.

Further Reading

Goffman E 1968a (1961) Asylums: essays in the social situation of mental patients and other inmates. Penguin, Harmondsworth

Goffman's original text should be essential reading for any nurse. It is not the most simple of books to read first time around but the introduction provides a sound overview of his thesis and the first chapter on the inmate world helps in developing an understanding of the impact of power in the caring services.

Goodall C 1995 Is disability any business of nurse education? Nurse Education Today 15(5): 325–327

This article challenges a medical model of disability that is diagnosis based, individualistic and necessarily tragic. Goodall also criticises the present politically correct social model and describes an 'interface model' which centres on the daily experience of disabled people. In so doing he mounts a direct assault on the labelling process by addressing ways in which an oppressive environment can become less restrictive and more caring.

Sontag S 1978 Illness as metaphor. Penguin, Harmondsworth
This short and very readable book provides an alternative view of the world of illness and its links with deviance. It is of particular value to nurses in that it challenges some of the commonly held beliefs about the impact of illness on the individual.

References

Becker H 1963 Outsiders: studies in the sociology of deviance. Free Press, New York

Berger P, Luckman T 1971 The social construction of reality. Penguin, Harmondsworth

Blumer H 1962 Society as symbolic interaction. In: Rose A (ed) Human behavior and social processes: an interactionist approach. Routledge and Kegan Paul, London, pp 179–192

Blumer H 1966 Sociological implications of the thoughts of George Herbert Mead. American Journal of Sociology March: 535–548

Blumer H 1969 Symbolic interactionism: perspective and method. Prentice Hall, Englewood Cliffs, NJ

Edgerton R 1967 The cloak of competence: stigma in the lives of the mentally retarded. University of California Press, Berkeley

Giddens A 1984 The constitution of society. Polity Press, Cambridge

Goffman E 1968a Asylums: essays on the social situation of mental patients and other inmates. Penguin, Harmondsworth

Goffman E 1968b Stigma: notes on the management of spoiled identity. Penguin, Harmondsworth

Goodall C 1995 Is disability any business of nurse education? Nurse Education Today 15(5): 325–327

Gove W 1980 Labelling and mental illness: a critique. In: Gove W (ed) The labelling of deviance. Sage, London

Hewison A 1995 Nurses power in interactions with patients. Journal of Advanced Nursing 21: 75–82

Johnson M, Webb C 1995 Rediscovering unpopular patients: the concept of social judgement. Journal of Advanced Nursing 21: 75–82

Lemert E 1967 Human deviance, social problems and social control. Prentice Hall, NJ

Prior P 1995 Surviving psychiatric institutionalisation: a case study. Sociology of Health and Illness 17: 651–667

Rosenhan D 1973 On being sane in unsane places. Science 179, 250–258

Scheff 1966 Being Mentally Ill: A Sociological Theory. Aldine, Chicago

Schneider J, Conrad P 1981 Medical and sociological typologies: the case of epilepsy. Social Science and Medicine 15: 211–219

Stockwell F 1972 The unpopular patient. Royal College of Nursing, London

Zeitlin I 1973 Rethinking sociology: a critique of contemporary theory. Prentice Hall, Englewood Cliffs, NJ

THE SOCIAL CONTEXT OF NURSING

Key concepts

- Breaking the rules
- Becoming a patient
- The unpopular patient
- Institutionalisation
- Whistle blowing

- Generalism in nursing
- Professionalisation
- Multiskilling
- Multidisciplinary work
- Nursing specialisms in a changing economy of care
- Normalisation

- The doctor–patient relationship
- Rules in nursing
- Power and social control

- Training and education of nurses
- Trade Unionism
- Profession or craft?
- Social model v medical model
- Vocationalism v professionalism

Having laid some foundations of sociology in the preceding two sections, Section 3 moves into the sociology of nursing and health care, and looks afresh at the ways in which we work with people, whether they are colleagues or clients. The emphasis is on relationships between nurses and colleagues and between nurses and patients/clients. Wider aspects of power and professionalism are considered through a review of key sociological studies that have examined the ways in which the 'tasks' of nursing can lack benefit to the client or patient.

A slight move in direction is taken as Section 3 ends with an overview of professionalisation and the significance of changes in working patterns which require the nurse to work in partnership with many other professionals: the multidisciplinary role. A particular emphasis is the mapping of the nurse as professional, the nature of the relationship between the various 'professional' groups allied to medicine and the linkage between health-care and social-care arenas.

Nurses, Clients and Power

Martin Johnson

Key concepts

- Nurses are weak in relation to other groups
- Clients often fail to exploit their power
- Goals of care are based on a balance of power
- Power is complex
- The effects of power cannot always be seen

This chapter is about the relationship between nurses and their clients and the power that holds it together. It also considers some of the wider issues of power as an aspect of professionalism in order to link with Chapter 9. In particular we will examine how it is that nursing care, as currently conceived, can effectively 'disempower' clients despite the official desire to increase their independence. The place of nurses in relation to other professionals is examined briefly; this is developed further in Chapter 9. We then look at the ways in which nurses and clients negotiate, and sometimes collide, in seeking to influence events. In particular, we examine the strategies that clients and their nurses may use to access power and achieve objectives. Sometimes these goals are less in tune with client preferences than we would like to think. The chapter concludes with a discussion of particular views of power which, though not new, have perhaps been neglected in nursing literature.

The Concept of Power

Although we all probably imagine that we have an idea of what power means, a concrete definition is usually found wanting.

The great British philosopher Bertrand Russell (1938) argued that it is 'the production of intended effects' which seems reasonable. If we want to achieve something and we can make it happen, then we must have had the 'power' to do so. Unfortunately this view now seems rather oversimplified. Our actions and those of others may also have unintended effects that illustrate our 'power'. For example, when nurses put on a uniform it may not be directly to create obedience in their clients, but it often has this type of effect, and of course the nurse's power to influence the client's behaviour increases accordingly.

Both philosophers and sociologists have wrestled with clarifying the concept of power. One of the most widely respected of these, who is seen as both sociologist and philosopher, is Steven Lukes (1974). His and other theories of power are examined at the end of this chapter, but to give a flavour of the complexity he describes power as 'ineradicably value-dependent' and 'essentially contested'. By this he means that Russell and others had failed to take into account the history and culture that people bring to the use and the understanding of power.

Nurses and Power

Many books address the question of the power of the nurse but it may be fair to say that this is often in the context of leadership and the simplistic Russell-type view prevails. Bryan Turner (1987), however, makes the important point that, in the context of work, nurses are for the most part instruments of the power of at least one other occupational group: the doctors. This builds upon the earlier, but still very relevant analysis by Eliot Freidson (1970) in which he argues that all occupations whose work is essentially 'medical' in character cannot fail to be subordinate in authority and responsibility to the medical profession. Turner goes on to illustrate how it is that what dentists are allowed to do is very tightly controlled by the medical profession. In this 'control by limitation' dentists, despite a six-year training, are confined to work on the teeth, and may practise wider 'surgery' only under strict control. Turner shows how other occupations with claims to manage illness, such as the clergy and practitioners of **alternative therapy** are controlled largely by 'exclusion'. The excluding profession maintains a register of legally licensed practitioners to which only the properly qualified are admitted. Turner argues that the strategy through which the medical profession controls nurses is by 'subordination'. Taking an historical perspective he seems to mean that, partly by means of their status as educated men, doctors successfully convinced not only a willing public and government, but nurses themselves (less-well-educated women), that medicine rightfully controls all medical work and that much of this that is mundane should be delegated to 'inferior' occupations whilst physicians and surgeons retain overall 'responsibility'. If this analysis is correct, we must conclude that much of what nurses do will be, whether they realise it or not, in pursuit of medically desired objectives. This view casts doubt on the validity of much of the rhetoric on the nursing process which speaks of nurses and clients agreeing mutually acceptable goals for which the nurse will be accountable (Roper et al 1996).

Another dimension to the question of nurses' power base is that they are also subordinated to another group: the professional health service managers who increasingly have business-related objectives. Nurses have begun to sense an important constraint to the development of autonomy in the face of targets set by managers who, for the most part, are not nurses. Overall, the resultant picture is one where Conrad (1979) feels that nurses can best be described as 'captive professionals'.

Clients and Power

A good deal of the language of the last decade has been in terms of client (or patient) empowerment. Even the increasing use of the term client for health service consumers reflects this trend. The term client generally refers to a person who purchases services directly from a professional. In the **private health sector** this could increasingly describe the situation accurately even though the majority of clients are still paying via a once-removed bureaucracy such as an insurance plan (rather than with cash). However, the word client has become popular as it intends to convey a more equal relationship between the recipient of care and the provider. How much this equality is the case in reality is of great interest. This section examines the ways in which clients could, and sometimes do, exploit what power is available and how, perhaps more commonly, they comply with nursing and medical goals.

Work

At first glance, work has little to do with the client's experiences of health care, especially if we accept Parsons' (1951) view of the sick role in which ill people are exempted from their normal work and responsibilities provided that they want to get well and comply with medical instructions. On closer analysis, however, work is a key source of power and influence for clients. Strauss et al (1982) suggest that using a 'sociology of work' perspective can illuminate much in the social relations between clients and their carers in hospital. They identify the place of 'work' carried out by clients in hospital in providing a basis for negotiation on other dimensions of social relations. Indeed they note that the staff's opinion of clients may depend on the nature of the work that they (clients) are prepared to do. Strauss et al (1982) identify as work many activities which take place in hospitals and in which clients are involved. They suggest that some work is officially recognised in the hospital division of labour, such as diabetics injecting their own insulin. Other work is not so recognised and may include clients reporting mistakes or deterioration in their client colleagues. Of particular interest is the interpersonal dimension in which Strauss et al identify clients' endurance of painful or uncomfortable procedures as work through which the client can then negotiate in other domains. Another area of work that if not done properly gets clients 'into trouble with staff', is the case of the very ill person who knows she or he is dying. Strauss et al suggest that the client is expected to do (unrecognised) work to maintain reasonable control over reactions which might be excessively disturbing of the staff's work, or disruptive of other clients' poise (see Case study 8.1).

This unrecognised work has been called **sentimental work** (Strauss et al 1982) or **emotional labour** (James 1989). James' paper analyses the notion of largely unpaid and 'invisible' emotional work from the viewpoint of the female health worker. She argues from an explicitly feminist (and arguably Marxist) perspective that women are socialised into providing unpaid labour without which the elite aspects of care, such as medical work, could not take place. Strauss et al (1982), however, focus on the role of the client in the ward division of labour illustrating that they too contribute an untold amount of emotional labour (what they term sentimental work). They argue further (although certainly not from a Marxist perspective) that this work contributes to the development of the patient–client relationship or its deterioration. It seems particularly relevant today to examine the nature of patient work in all or any of its forms, since independence or 'self care' are increasingly aspects of both nursing and government ideology. The part this work (or its absence) plays in the management of human relations and the use and abuse of power are examined again later.

Case study 8.1

Consider the case of Nick, who was terminally ill. Nick had lung cancer which had spread seriously. He had agreed to radiation therapy which both he and nursing staff knew was probably futile. Nick was able to get away with disturbing a ward report to get medication, usually an unacceptable behaviour, perhaps because he was careful in his control of the more emotive consequences of his diagnosis. Publically, he did not challenge the decision of the doctors that he should have more treatment.

This insight is useful because it also identifies client work as a source of power, or a legitimate negotiating resource. It is a source of clients' control over their social situation; in this case getting his medication early. It also shows that on the 'big issues' he was relatively powerless.

Complaining

Another opportunity to exploit the limited power available to clients is the complaint. Much complaining in hospital is 'off stage' and out of earshot of the nurses. It happens in the day rooms and toilet areas and health professionals often have little knowledge of it.

What is known comes largely from the work of sociologists like Benyon (1987) who have been clients and, when well enough, have realised that they could learn much from observing and recording the insights available as opportunistic participant observers. Benyon noted the 'grumbling' of clients in a surgical ward which was not meant to be heard by the staff. Such behaviour helps to relieve frustration and gives a degree of social support to otherwise vulnerable persons in the anxiety-laden atmosphere, especially of the surgical ward.

Some formal complaints are made, however, and can present a threat to nurses who may perceive their image of competence to be under attack. The problem for the client is often the judgement of the moment when a complaint really is the best course, in a context in which complaining can be labelled as 'difficult behaviour'. According to English & Morse (1988), in their ethnography of 'difficult' elderly clients, nurses said that 'complaining clients made them feel they could never do anything right' (1988:28). Clearly clients do complain both about day-to-day concerns like the tea being too hot, or too cold. On the other hand, clients can be motivated to 'risk' their social reputation by complaining, especially where they feel that they have nothing to lose because they feel that their social reputation is already damaged. They are, as Goffman (1968) would put it, 'stigmatised' or 'with spoiled identity'. Sometimes the criticism is more personal as in Case study 8.2.

The case study illustrates a client exploiting a localised complaint mechanism to influence events as they affect him. Objectively speaking this is legitimate, but is nevertheless seen as a course of last resort by many clients. It also points out the accountability that student nurses are subject to. Despite being only a relatively inexperienced student, Paula was directly accountable both to the staff nurses and to the client for the care that she gave. This illustrates the way in which much discussion of accountability, as a thing that goes hand in hand with autonomy, may be misguided. The rhetoric of professionalism is that with accountability comes autonomy; however, this sort of example shows that being answerable for actions (accountable) in this potentially painful way is rather a feature of the least powerful of health-care professionals than of the elite, such as the consultant physician, the clinical nurse specialist, or the university lecturer. To return to Freidson's (1970) brilliant analysis (which nurses have largely ignored in their own claims to professional status), true professionalism means 'legitimate organised autonomy' and this is

Case study 8.2

Charles, who had very serious chronic airways obstruction, and was constantly weak from lack of oxygen and carbon dioxide excess, had apparently lost confidence in Paula, one of the junior nurses on the ward. Charles asked the staff nurse to arrange for his care to be carried out by someone else as he felt that Paula was slow and clumsy. At one level he was expressing a legitimate preference if, indeed, Paula had caused him previous discomfort. At another level he must have assumed that 'reporting her' to a staff nurse might be a sanction both for her and an example to others.

Consider the view that he had power over both the staff nurse and Paula, at that and subsequent moments. Charles had long since given up trying to be popular; his condition of chronic airflow limitation was too discomforting and frightening to allow him to keep up appearances of 'niceness'. So in complaining he had less to lose, and something to gain. At least he did not 'suffer' Paula's care which in his eyes was inadequate to his needs at that time. Such a tactic illustrates how clients can resort to conflict if necessary.

not the same thing as accountability as the ward nurse experiences it. In other words, autonomy really means not being accountable in any meaningful way to the client.

Exchange

Another attempt to restore the balance of power between nurse and client is the exchange of services and, to a limited extent, of gifts. Officially discouraged from accepting 'substantial' gifts, nurses are often offered small tokens of appreciation by clients. Sweets, chocolates and tights seem to be popular. Janice Morse (1989), identifying the importance of gift-giving in the anthropological literature, suggests that the giving of care by nurses creates a further imbalance in an already unequal relationship between nurse and client. Clients commonly wish to reciprocate by giving 'gifts' to attempt to equalise things. Although this notion may seem at first sight relatively inconsequential, the point is that the 'gift relationship' is a concept of some importance in the understanding of service relationships such as exist between clients and nurses. Malcolm Johnson (1975), drawing on Marcel Mauss, argues that the giving and receiving of gifts is symbolic rather than economic. It is a confirmation of reciprocity that exists between individuals and groups. Johnson's thesis is that the elderly are frequently disempowered in these terms by being systematically excluded from the possibility of reciprocity, for example by being rendered poor and socially isolated.

Such a notion is one possible explanation of the weak power-base of clients. Generally the range of 'gifts' available is small. Indeed it may be that the offering of such relatively insubstantial items as sweets is a modest attempt to fill the gap left by the minimal opportunity for a truly balanced exchange of services or other 'gifts'. Where 'client work' in the terms of Strauss et al (1982) can be seen as an aspect of this 'gift exchange' idea, it becomes clear how those who cannot offer even this will be seriously disempowered in their presentation of themselves as 'socially worthwhile'. 'Exchange theory' has been influential in most of the social and behavioural sciences. One key idea apart from the giving of services and actual gift artefacts is that individuals also bring aspects of their background, culture and class into any relationship, all of which helps to bring either balance or disorder to social interaction. Simplistically therefore, young university-educated nurses might have little in common with the elderly retired bus conductor, and so will spend little enough time interacting with this person except at a very instrumental level of 'routine care'. Although studies show that this can determine some aspects of care (Stockwell 1972), Kelly & May (1982) argued that such a view fails to recognise the true complexity of human interaction in specific circumstances. In one study, for example, one elderly man was failing to comply with medication, smoked despite being an oxygen user, was quite elderly and seemed to meet the criteria for being a 'social problem' (Johnson & Webb 1995). As it happened this person, whom exchange theory would have predicted to have been unpopular and with little influence over his care, was quite the reverse. He was able, through his manifest bubbly personality and stoic acceptance of discomforts, to win respect and concessions from the nursing staff.

Conflict

Whereas the 'gift' relationship can be seen as an attempt to grasp some sort of influence in a socially acceptable way, often such an agreeable approach fails and the client may have exhausted or ignored the formal channels of complaint. It is probably true to say that texts on nursing care emphasise consensus and mutual goal setting in planning care. Conflict is not seriously considered as an aspect of 'nursing models' which purport to explain and predict client behaviour and nursing care. An example is that in Roper et al (1996) which, although produced by British academics, has a good deal in common with its American counterparts. In contrast to 'nursing theory', much important sociological theory has identified conflict as a fundamental concept. According to Lukes (1974) the presence of conflict is a key test of power in any relationship but should not be seen as the only test. Conflict has been seen as a struggle between competing classes or groups in society. Here we will discuss conflict in a fairly small-scale way as representing the struggle between individual clients and health professionals for the achievement of day-to-day goals rather than political objectives.

In an analysis of the strategies of clients in an alcohol treatment facility, Fineman (1991) presents categories at variance with the prevailing consensus view of professional–client relations. He argues that clients frequently resort to the subversive to achieve their own, rather than the health professionals', goals. Under a category of 'manipulation' he lists 'sabotage', where clients deliberately frustrate the professionals' intentions. One strategy might be failing to turn up for group meetings, being late for therapy sessions or failing to supply specimens for investigation. Think about the Case study 8.3 which is taken from practice.

Case study 8.3

Bob was a very ill client with alcoholic cirrhosis of the liver and tuberculosis from living rough. He was acutely ill, but was able to get the less experienced nurses to give his sedative medications earlier than the prescription sheet allowed. This was because they seemed afraid that if he did not get his own way some of the time, he would fail to stay on his side when he was turned and so the staff would be blamed for failing to keep him off his pressure areas. He knew that they were nervous of being 'accountable' for the worsening of his pressure areas.

Bob is a good example of a client who has 'nothing to lose' by being openly in conflict with the nursing staff. He would make promises that if left in bed all morning, he would get up for an hour in the afternoon, but later nurses would find that he had told the afternoon shift that he had already been exhausted by the morning staff getting him out.

Under a second category of 'working the system' Fineman lists 'doctor shopping', seeking undeserved services, and provoking fights among the staff. Doctor-shopping amounts to recruiting multiple staff members to work toward contradictory ends.

Compliance

It would be wrong to overestimate the ability of clients to utilise these strategies in achieving their own goals in defiance of those of the nursing and medical staff. Very frequently clients will hold out for the unimportant, such as an extra cup of tea or the right not to be bathed first thing in the morning, only to comply with the health professionals' wishes on the 'big' issues, such as whether to undergo uncomfortable and even dangerous treatments. Freidson (1970) drew attention to the theoretical point of great relevance here. There are objective differences in perspective between the client and the professional (in this case the nurse). Therefore, whatever the client may do to impose their view, any success erodes claims to professionalism.

Frequently nursing and other health occupations will recruit extra-professional support for their intentions, such as appeals to relatives. Many people would take no issue with Parsons' (1951) view that **compliance** with medical instructions is in everyone's interests. The study by Waterworth & Luker (1990) showed that, at least in one Liverpool hospital, many clients were keen to 'toe the line' because they saw no reason to be involved in decisions about their care. They assumed that the professions knew best and that, in any case, they felt vulnerable, like being in a dentist's chair. That is to say, they perceive a physical or emotional threat of discomfort which renders them compliant. Nurses, like dentists, have a wide range of very uncomfortable or embarrassing procedures at their disposal, a point we shall expand later.

Interestingly, most medical research literature on compliance sees it uncritically as something to be achieved in societal interests. Sociologists on the other hand have taken the opposite view with perhaps a most ardent (if polemical) advocate Ivan Illich (1976) arguing that compliance with medical care is dangerous to health on a number of levels. His polemic 'Limits to Medicine (Medical Nemesis)' is essential reading in order to develop a really critical appreciation of the role of medicine in health care.

Before examining nurses' power in more detail, you may like to reflect on the notion of client labelling which can be seen as a key aspect of the maintenance of nursing power.

Activity 8.1	Thinking about social judgement Write down two examples from your own experience in which clients have seemed 'unpopular'. Why do you think this was, and how did you and your colleagues behave toward them? Recall from your own experience clients who 'broke the rules' but still remained popular with the nursing staff. Later in this chapter we will look briefly at this issue and you may compare your experiences with the points made here.

We will now give some attention to the ways in which nurses exploit their privileged and powerful position.

Nurses' Power and the Client's Response

A wide range of strategies are available to health professionals in general, and nurses in particular, which enable the effective control of clients in the direction of professional goals. Here we will discuss a selection of those which may perhaps seem controversial or that you may not have thought of as aspects of social control. Think critically about the suggestions made in relation to your own practice experiences.

Control of Information

Nurses control most of the information flow in relation to the care of clients. They maintain the main record systems, control telephone and other information media in most if not all clinical areas, and even decide who may and may not enter clinical areas and the times when this will be allowed. They frequently act as gatekeeper to other professionals, notably the doctors. The 'Sisters Office', or its equivalent, is a place where personal and clinical information is centralised under the control of specific nursing staff. Given their structural control over communications, nurses are also well versed in the arts of secrecy. David Field (1989) argues that despite some changes from the systematic lying to virtually all clients about serious diagnoses, a good deal of information of concern to the very ill client is still kept hidden in a 'silent conspiracy'. Clients are still deprived of information about their prognosis whatever progress has been made on the front of openness about diagnosis. Of course it can be argued that this is done for the best of reasons, that the paternalism here is justified on the grounds of saving clients unnecessary anxiety and allowing hope where none may be possible. Whether or not it is finally in the client's interests, this strategy emphasises the power of the doctors compared to the client. It can only be concluded that nurses collude substantially in this. Given that nurses operate in a mode of only guarded release of information they are in a position which inevitably disempowers their clients. They manage the uncertainty clients have about their future.

Depersonalisation

More controversially, it can be argued that nurses maintain a strategy of disempowerment of their clients which, although not deliberate as such, has evolved to play a major place in the achievement of medical and increasingly managerial objectives in health service provision. One of the tactics in this strategy is depersonalisation. Goffman (1968) and others have noted that excessive routine, wearing of night clothes at most times of the day, deprivation of usual privacy and the systematic changing of daily routine from the personal to the institutional are key factors in the causation of patterns of behaviour which engage the compliance of 'inmates' for the nurses. Whatever the rhetoric of individualised care, many of these features remain in mainstream hospital practice. Furthermore, the procedures for the delivery of 'individualised care' have contributed systematically to the collection and centralisation of sensitive patient data in nursing process kardexes, care plans and computerised patient administration systems.

Humiliation

Even more controversial is the accusation that a key tactic in the process of disempowerment (or the engagement of compliance) is **humiliation**. Littlewood (1991) argues that historically nurses have taken more than a necessary interest in the physical body of the client, focusing in particular on the bowel. People are asked in public to describe their recent evacuations, are asked to defaecate into bedpans and present the resulting matter for scrutiny, and are regularly and routinely asked to submit to insertion of gloved fingers and other items into the rectum. Bowel habit becomes a matter for public discourse in a way completely at variance with the usual social conventions. Even routine bowel habit takes place in a toilet usually much more public than the nurses would choose for themselves. Such facts could be seen to be matters of clinical necessity (although we doubt it), but the fundamental point is that they are very embarrassing. This embarrassment helps to give the client a very different status from the nurse; indeed, the nurse's privacy in such matters is well protected by way of special 'staff only' toilets which help to preserve both the dignity and status of the staff.

Activity 8.2

Thinking about status

Think of other examples from your day-to-day work that create a difference in status between you and your clients. Why do these differences exist?

Social Judgement

In the box above we have alluded to the social reputation of the client and the nurse. Labelling, or the process of **social judgement**, is another dimension of the disempowerment of clients by nurses in the health-care context. First described substantially by Roth (1972) and Stockwell (1972), the process of labelling people as 'good', 'bad', 'popular' or 'unpopular' has been examined more closely from an interpretive perspective by Kelly & May (1982) and Johnson & Webb (1995). Generally it can be argued that most clients and their nurses are aware of the differing social judgements that each makes of the other, and that this viewpoint can become part of the bargain for co-operation in achieving goals of care. Often, staff views of a client vary, indeed they may be renegotiated by the client in relation to new 'evidence' or behaviour. The 'official' or dominant view of a client can be an important backdrop to the type of decision made about their care and can even play a part in important moral decisions. Some nurses report having to 'like people secretly' because they do not feel ready to challenge the prevailing view of a client. Nurses even adopt strategies of secret caring to 'compensate' or advocate for the client they feel is unfairly seen in a bad light (Johnson & Webb 1995). It is important, however, to avoid the assumption that certain characteristics necessarily lead to 'unpopularity'. Like access to 'power', many factors are involved and there is much that depends on the social context of the time, place and people involved.

These strategies are illustrations of the source of nursing power in relation to the client and it is important to remember that in reality more factors come into play. You may be able to identify others, or you may feel that the view portrayed here is rather pessimistic and sees health professionals in too sinister a light. The provision of excellent care probably does depend on professionals having a certain amount of authority to act and to make decisions based on their extensive professional knowledge. This view is now examined in more detail, by discussing this 'functional' view of health professional power and two of its competitors.

Theoretical Issues

You will recall that we can see power as a very complex notion. This section reviews some key views of power to examine their ability to illuminate some of the issues and examples discussed earlier. Russell's (1938) view of the production of intended effects is clearly too simple. Because many clients are socialised to accept the authority of the professional, nurses may be more powerful than they intend to be. A small study by Waterworth & Luker (1990) illustrates how many clients do not wish or expect to be involved in decisions about their care, but the explanation probably lies in the powerful socialisation to accept professional authority to which, throughout their lives, they have been subject.

Power as Functional

Nursing authors have realised the importance of power. Benner (1984) is widely influential and is arguably more credible than some other nursing theory because it is drawn from direct observation of practice. In her book she argues consistently that experience and reflection combine to produce expertise and the ability to wield clinical power in an 'excellent' way. The following direct quote from Benner's research illustrates her viewpoint fairly well:

Reflection point 8.1

'The nurses who took part in this study have offered us glimpses of the nature of the power that resides in caring. They have used their power to empower their patients – not to dominate, coerce, or control them. But this relationship is highly contextual. To empower, nurses sometimes border on coercion as they coach and prompt the patient to engage in painful tasks that patients would not readily undertake on their own. The difference between empowerment and domination can be understood only if the nurse–patient relationship and the situation are understood. Caring out of context will always be controversial, because caring is local, specific, and individual.'
    (Benner 1984:209)

Analyse this quote and try to decide which kind of view of power Benner has. Keep it in mind when we look at theories of power from the wider philosophical and sociological literature. Does it have anything in common with Parsons? Compare it with the views of Foucault and Lukes later in this chapter.

Parsons

Parsons (1951) viewed socialisation as necessary to a functioning social system. Through the media of education, religion, the law and medicine, Parsons saw the exercise of power merely as a proper tool of social control to avoid anarchy and inefficiency. Power, in a later work by Parsons (1963), is simply a system resource (not unlike money) to be used, preferably by those properly so authorised (professionals) to return the sick to 'normal functioning'. Parsons saw professional power as derived by legitimate consensus and therefore necessarily good. This view of power could be described as 'power to'. Parsons does not see any possibility of the use of power for illegitimate purposes, and so from a modern perspective we must see this view as perhaps too conservative. For example in December 1986 nurse Yuen How Choy was convicted of raping a woman at her home after pretending to examine her. He had also abused his privileged position in 1972 by sedating a woman in order to have sex with her. Inexplicably the United Kingdom Central Council (UKCC) restored this nurse to the nursing register, when Mr Choy got referees to say that he was otherwise of good character (Nursing Times

1996). Such cases provoke anger and dismay among nurses, politicians and the public, but the key point is that from time to time health professionals, including nurses, do abuse power in a way that Parsons' assumptions about professionals being moral leaders of the community would deny. Not only this, but self-regulation – a key attribute of a profession – can sometimes be seen manifestly to fail to protect the public. Over the past few years, examples of this abuse of power have emerged from the Special Hospital Service. In a recent book Adams (1997) describes incidents of physical abuse by staff towards their clients that clearly have no place in a caring environment.

Whistleblowing

The UKCC for Nursing, Midwifery and Health Visiting issue a Code of Professional Conduct which applies to every nurse whose name appears on the Professional Register. In relation to the accountability clause in the Code Orr (1995) writes:

> 'The Code seeks to state important principles which should guide practice. The interests of the public and the patient or client are seen as paramount and the practitioner should recognise that these interests must predominate over those of the nurse. In addition, each practitioner must be personally and professionally accountable in such a manner as to respect the primacy of the interests of the client.'
>   (Orr 1995:51)

The inference taken from this quotation would suggest that any nurse who witnesses or knows about malpractice should report this to her or his line manager or to the professional statutory body – in short to blow the whistle on nursing, medical or ancillary colleagues who wilfully neglect their duty in respect of a patient or client. In the past many abuses previously referred to have gone undetected because of management or peer group pressure to turn a blind eye. Since the inception of the Code of Professional Conduct and the increasing popularity of patient/client advocacy schemes, particularly in the related fields of mental health and learning disability, more nurses are coming forward to expose abuse and malpractice. However, because of the complex power relationships which exist within a heirarchical and bureaucratic organisation such as the health service, it takes courage to blow the whistle. Notable people such as Graham Pink, a Stockport nurse who mounted a vigorous campaign against what he saw as a poor care environment for his elderly patients, failed in his bid to receive whole-hearted support for his actions. Clearly he suffered personally and professionally for taking the action he did. In other cases it often rests with the media to expose malpractice, and a number of instances are on record where prosecution has followed such exposure.

<table>
<tr><td>**Activity 8.3**</td><td>Blowing the whistle

You are on day duty in a ward for elderly people and you see a nursing colleague roughly handle a patient who has been incontinent whilst sitting in his chair. Later in the day you notice severe bruising to the patient's right arm. Having witnessed the earlier incident and recalling it was the same arm that your colleague had taken hold of when removing the patient so roughly from his chair, reflect on your professional and moral responsibilities in this case.</td></tr>
</table>

To recapitulate, Parsons' (and arguably Benner's) view, in assuming experience and expertise are necessary and sufficient conditions for practice which is entirely in clients' interests, may be insufficiently cognisant of dangers of malpractice. Parsons' view may seem dated, but something like it underlies much paternalistic thinking among health professionals and it could be said to be an influence behind concepts of 'general management', efficiency and effectiveness, and the current fashion for educating for purpose. The view is flawed because it assumes that each professional is altruistic and generally acts primarily in clients' interests alone.

Michel Foucault

A more complex view of power which has received relatively little attention in nursing literature is that of Michel Foucault (1991). As with Parsons, a brief introduction to his ideas risks injustice to them, but his perspective is so challenging (especially to health professionals) that it is worthy of some discussion. He takes a historical approach to the evolution of ideas and social relations, examining in his various books, psychiatry, medicine, legal systems and the theory of knowledge. He notes that in order to wield power over people, those in authority used to have to use torture, restraint, imprisonment and incarceration to control those in society who presented some kind of threat to the dominant order. His evidence is indisputable. Some of his text makes very emotive reading, such as his graphic account of hanging, drawing and quartering. In relation to the health professions he shows how, at first, lepers were seen as a threat to society so that they were excluded from 'society' by incarceration. Later, as leprosy became less important, other previously well tolerated groups were marginalised and incarcerated, such as the mentally ill and, in the nineteenth century, the poor.

Foucault is not arguing that modern health professionals, nor even prison officers, undertake these approaches to the exercise of power. Rather he argues that over time we have subtly absorbed such events into our collective consciousness as the legitimation for our preparedness to be subject to the authority of others. Now, those in authority can usually control the behaviour of others by much more subtle means but which have, in their history, these brutal physical methods to which, were it ever necessary, those in power could resort. These gentler but just as effective means he describes collectively as 'The Gaze'.

Hierarchical Observation

Through what Foucault (1991) calls surveillance, information is collected about those to be subjugated and controlled. Systems are developed (for which read the nursing process) more effectively to collect and distribute this information among those who may need it. Foucault observed that the ideal prison (called the panopticon) is one where all the inmates can be seen by just one officer, not unlike the 'Nightingale' ward in a hospital. As subjects become accustomed to their position in this social order, they can even be relied upon to undertake self-surveillance, which emphasises Foucault's point that power is as much given up by the subjects as taken by the powerful.

Normalising Judgement

Powerful people, in this case nurses, monitor the behaviour of their clients, executing penalties for infringements of acceptable behaviour and, most importantly, controlling the social reputation of their clients. It is in this way that the opinions of the 'powerful' nurse carry weight in decisions about the client's future. Detailed knowledge of activity, speech and particularly the body is maintained, with the potential for humiliation being exploited at every opportunity when control is necessary. With this in mind, Littlewood's (1991) thesis on the importance to nurses of surveillance of bowel habit (and other intimate functions) begins to have some explanation.

The Examination

This is the ritual collection of appropriate data, but it also acts as the symbolic act of disempowerment. Just as executions in the middle ages were undertaken with the subject naked, specifically to enhance the humiliation (if this were possible), the ritual of nakedness and detailed examination of the body and (increasingly) of the personality is maintained. It is particularly important to the idea that it is only the client that submits to 'the examination'. Health professionals go to considerable lengths to avoid their private circumstances becoming known to clients as this would provide access to 'power' for clients and would erode claims to professionalism.

Foucault's view of power is nothing if not interesting. He defied requests to define power absolutely, preferring it to be seen as in a diffuse conjoint relationship with knowledge, which as can be seen is integral to the maintenance of, or rather access to, power. He argues that power is as much given up by the weak as taken by the strong, and that all have access in certain contexts. There is no doubt that Michel Foucault is commonly regarded as taking an extreme view, polemical if you will, and is comparable to the influential (but equally extreme) Ivan Illich. On the other hand, nurses are vulnerable to criticism that their education in sociology, philosophy and other 'liberal' disciplines tends to be sanitised and rendered 'safe' for their consumption. Much that is of value in feminist discourse is marginalised for the same reason.

Steven Lukes

The last 'theorist' we will examine is Steven Lukes (1974). He argues that many conceptions of power are simplistic. He typifies the Russell view, for example, as one-dimensional. He suggests that such views as the production of intended effects are dependent on both the relevant actions and the effects being observable and able to be determined in advance. Any view in which power needs to be exercised presupposes a conflict of interests between the parties concerned. Such a view is not common in the health professions as most practitioners argue that they only act in the interests of the client. A second approach to the analysis of power would be a two-dimensional view. Here, one face of power would be based in the observable actions and effects of decisions based on power. The second face of this more complex view of power is what Lukes loosely calls 'bias'. It is the extent to which a person or group consciously or unconsciously creates obstructions to openness. Here he seems to suggest that together with open use of control measures goes a more sinister, less open form of power analogous to coercion. He notes that this view of power still has conflict at its roots, and that the 'bias' or coercive element can best be revealed by discovering 'grievances' (complaints) that the disempowered may hold; however, he remains unsatisfied by this 'extended behavioural' view of power.

Because he is dissatisfied with the 'individualistic' nature of the previous views of power, Lukes proposes a three-dimensional view of power that incorporates a systemic or organisational dimension. The key aspect that he adds to his view of power can be illustrated as follows. He draws upon a Marxist concept analogous to hegemony to argue that people make their own history but they are not fully in control of it. They do not choose the circumstances of their birth or, to a large extent, their socialisation. Rather, the extra dimension is the sense in which power can be used to shape the very needs, wants and preferences of those we would subjugate. This is particularly apposite in the analysis of health care where clients' needs and wants are primarily determined by health professionals. To put it another way, health and health care are defined by health professionals who then wholly control access (or not) to it.

Lukes' (1974) radical model of power goes beyond that of Parsons to examine what the exercise of power prevents people from doing and even thinking. The model is 'radical' because it makes the assumption that individuals or groups have responsibility for the exercise (or not) of their power. This view of power has a certain appeal in health care because it brings into focus what in ethics is called the acts and omissions doctrine. This states that just as much responsibility attaches to a decision not to act as is attached to a decision to act in a given circumstance. This may be as simple as failing to make a contrary opinion known about the plan of care for a client.

Case study 8.4 On a medical ward-round, Bill, an elderly man with a severe arthritic condition of the feet was authorised to go home at the earliest convenience because his medication was now stabilised and no further treatment was possible. He did not live far away, but could walk only with considerable discomfort. It was late afternoon and the newly qualified staff nurse knew that it was too late to order an ambulance for that day. She had the option of authorising a hospital taxi, but she decided that, since Bill would probably manage without one once he got home, she would ask him to find his own way home by bus or pay for a taxi himself. This decision is routine enough, but became problematic when she asked a male staff nurse (who did not really agree) to tell Bill the decision because 'he'll take it better from a man'. This second staff nurse did tell him and, with a little persuasion and the offer of a wheelchair to the door, he agreed to go. The male staff nurse felt guilty at failing to act as an advocate for Bill and particularly for failing to discuss the issue more forcibly with the staff nurse. In this case 'loyalty' to the new staff nurse and a wish to maintain her confidence was, perhaps, misplaced when Bill's interests are considered.

According to Lukes (1974) view, the male staff nurse in Case study 8.4 is responsible (negatively if you like) for the situation of the client in having to find his own way home, perhaps in discomfort. By doing nothing, he is just as powerful in the interests of the hospital rather than the client. This can be even more important on issues arguably of greater consequence, such as whether to continue painful treatments for the very ill.

Summary

Power can be understood at many levels. The concept is complex, and yet examples can help to identify aspects such as social judgement, coercion, authority, humiliation, force, restraint, surveillance and incarceration which are among many devices we all use to access power in its many forms. This chapter has examined issues of the nature of power and the ways in which both clients and nurses may gain access to it in order to influence events. It is certainly important to think more critically about such matters than may have been evident in nursing textbooks in the past. Power has consistently been seen as a legitimate professional resource based on knowledge and altruism of the nurse or doctor. Very frequently individual nurses and other health professionals clearly have clients' interests at heart. This may not, however, prevent them frustrating clients' preferences and goals because they are different from those the professionals have in mind. In order to discuss power at all, it is necessary to leave some of the conceptual complexities to one side, since the notion is so contested. What may be important, however, is to be aware of competing notions of power so that contemporary health-care practice may be analysed in relation to each. Observing the context of a client receiving an enema through the perspective of Michel Foucault produces a very different analysis than, say, Parsons or even Benner. Their views seem essentially flawed in the direction of experienced nurses always being 'nice people'. A critical appreciation of the sources of influence in health care is important. It has the implication for practice that nurses could more effectively act as advocates for their clients when necessary and, more importantly, will refrain from doing so when this is, in itself, a disempowering act.

Discussion questions

1. What are the main sources of influence that nurses have in relation to their clients?
2. What do you feel may be some of the reasons that patients in health care fail to be assertive in asking for information or making clear their views about treatment and care?
3. How much does the rather pessimistic view of Michel Foucault fit with your experiences as a health professional?

Further Reading

Johnson M 1997 Nursing power and social judgement. Ashgate, Aldershot

Developing substantially some of the ideas in this chapter, this book draws upon ethnographic research into the social context of decision making by nurses and others in health care. The book concentrates on how labelling forms a basis for the construction of nurses' and clients' relative use of and access to power.

Lawler J 1991 Behind the screens: nursing, somology, and the problems of the body. Churchill Livingstone, Melbourne

Joclyn Lawler's book is a very stimulating and readable account of her research as a participant observer in Australian hospitals. She recounts detailed examples of how it is that nurses 'manage' the bodies of those in their care, giving in my view a realistic picture of many 'taboo' areas for discussion. She takes a pragmatic approach to the method she uses, even 'deceiving' her respondents for some of the time. Overall, one gains a sense of reality from the book which many academics fail to portray.

Melia KM 1987 Learning and working: the occupational socialisation of student nurses. Tavistock, London

Kath Melia's influential and readable account of 40 'traditional' Registered General Nurses' experiences as student nurses is still a classic despite many of the organisational aspects of nursing education having changed in the ensuing decade.

Street AF 1992 Inside nursing: a critical ethnography of clinical nursing practice. State University of New York Press, New York

Annette Street's account of nursing practice (which, along with Lawler's is also Australian) has an explicitly feminist and critical-theory orientation. Like Lawler's book it helps to throw into stark relief the ways in which nurses and clients manage their different power bases.

References

Adams R 1997 The abuse of punishment. Macmillan, London, p116

Benner P 1984 Novice to expert: excellence and power in nursing. Addison-Wesley, Menlo Park, California

Benyon J 1987 Zombies in dressing gowns. In: McKeganey NP, Cunningham-Burley S (eds) Enter the sociologist, reflections on the practice of sociology. Avebury, Aldershot

Conrad P 1979 Types of medical social control. Sociology of Health and Illness 1(1): 1–11

English J, Morse JM 1988 The 'difficult' elderly patient: adjustment or maladjustment?, International Journal of Nursing Studies 25(1): 23–29

Field D 1989 Nursing the dying. Routledge, London

Fineman N 1991 The social construction of non-compliance: a study of health care and social service providers in everyday practice. Sociology of Health and Illness 13(3): 354–374

Foucault M 1991 Discipline and punish. Penguin, Harmondsworth

Freidson E 1970 Profession of medicine: a study of the sociology of applied knowledge. Dodd Mead, New York

Goffman E 1968 Asylums. Penguin, Harmondsworth

Illich I 1976 Limits to medicine. Marion Boyars, London

James N 1989 Emotional labour: skill and work in the social regulation of feelings. Sociological Review 37(1): 15–42

Johnson ML 1975 Old age and the gift relationship. New Society 13 March

Johnson M, Webb C 1995 Rediscovering unpopular patients: the concept of social judgement. Journal of Advanced Nursing 21: 466–475

Kelly MP, May D 1982 Good and bad patients: a review of the literature and a theoretical critique. Journal of Advanced Nursing 7: 147–156

Littlewood J 1991 Care and ambiguity: towards a concept of nursing. In: Holden P, Littlewood J (eds) Anthropology and nursing. Routledge, London

Lukes S 1974 Power: a radical view. Macmillan, London

Morse JM 1989 Gift-giving, reciprocity for care: gift giving in the patient–nurse relationship. Canadian Journal of Nursing Research 21(1): 33–45

Nursing Times 1996 Court orders UKCC to suspend reinstated rapist. Nursing Times 92(28): 5

Orr J 1995 Nursing accountability. In: Hunt G (ed) Whistleblowing in the Health Service, accountability, law and professional practice. Edward Arnold, London

Parsons T 1951 The social system. Free Press, Glencoe, Illinois

Parsons T 1963 Power and the social system. In: Lukes S (ed) Power. Blackwell, Oxford

Roper N, Logan W, Tierney AJ 1996 The elements of nursing. Churchill Livingstone, Edinburgh

Roth JA 1972 Some contingencies of the moral evaluation and control of clientele. American Journal of sociology 77: 839

Russell B 1938 The forms of power. In: Lukes S (ed) Power. Blackwell, Oxford

Stockwell F 1972 The unpopular patient. Royal College of Nursing, London

Strauss AL, Fagerhaugh S, Suczek B, Wiener C 1982 The work of hospitalised patients. Social Science and Medicine 16: 977–986

Turner BS 1987 Medical power and social knowledge. Sage, London

Waterworth S, Luker K 1990 Reluctant collaborators: do patients want to be involved in decisions concerning care? Journal of Advanced Nursing 15: 971–996

9 Professional and Educational Directions

Peter Birchenall

Key concepts

- Professionalism v vocationalism
- Generalism v specialism
- Social model v the medical model of care
- Multiskilling and shared learning in the primary health-care environment
- The growth of educational and professional development within the professions allied to medicine
- Multi-agency working
- The changing economy of care
- Interprofessional networking and the development of flexible learning strategies

This chapter considers the realities of nursing as a profession and the relationship between the nurse and other professionals. The notion of 'profession' will be considered in relation to nursing as a craft subject, and an examination of the education and training of nurses is carried out with a view to a greater understanding of where the family of nursing fits within the professional hierarchy. Possible future directions for nursing education and practice are reviewed taking account of such issues as National Vocational Qualifications (NVQ), all-graduate professional education and the implications of the move into higher education. This discussion leads into a debate surrounding the generic nurse and the possible diminishment of the specialist branches of nursing. Current theories of care are considered and linked to recent trends, particularly in adult nursing in relation to self-care and early discharge. The arguments also extend to learning disabilities and, in particular, theories surrounding normalisation and community care are discussed. Connections are made to Chapter 8 in respect of the power relationship between doctors and nurses and the use of authority and control. The nurse as a member of the multiprofessional team receives detailed consideration, and key elements of the nursing role are linked to educational and professional developments in professions allied to medicine (PAMs). The concluding part of the chapter explores nursing specialisms in a changing economy of care, moving across the four main branches through to the community specialisms and then onwards to the highly focused and specialist aspects of practice, such as stoma care, renal care, behavioural therapy, psychotherapy and neonatal care. Finally, the contentious notions of advanced and specialist practice are discussed.

Professionalism

The idea of 'professionalism' has exercised the minds of academics and others for many years and nursing is one of those occupational groups that makes a claim towards full recognition by society based on criteria that is said to reflect professional status, such as:

- self-regulation
- extension and advancement of a unique body of knowledge through established educational processes
- maintenance of a code of professional conduct underpinning a live register of practitioners
- admission to corporate membership based on strict standards of competence. These are attested by examinations and assessed experience, and a recognition that its practice must be for the benefit of the people it purports to serve, as well as that of its practitioners.

Literature on the subject of professionalism is extensive and it is not possible to do justice to all of it. For the purpose of this discussion two quotations illustrate the main elements of the professional role. The first is an early quote from the work of Imogene King:

> 'If nurses are to continue to function in a professional role, that role must be defined by the profession, and the educational programs must provide opportunities for socialisation into the profession.'
> (King 1981:2)

The second is from the literature on vocationalism:

> '... vocationalism should act as a mirror to reveal the true purpose of nursing and the current notion of nurses generally performing all activities,

required by patient or client, will require re-appraisal'.
(Warr 1996:267)

These quotations are selected for several reasons. First, there is an emphasis within the quote from Imogene King on the perception of professional role definition being inextricably bound up with education and training. Her second important emphasis is the overtly strong assumption that nursing is a professional activity into which practitioners are socialised. Warr in articulating the notion of what has become known as **vocationalism** provides a pointer to the rise in popularity of vocational qualifications for health carers and how these can be seen as a threat to the stability of nursing education. Vocationalism will be discussed later, but for now we occupy ourselves with the views proffered by Imogene King. It could be claimed by traditionalists that her arguments are central to any serious discussion concerning the activities of any occupational group which claims to be 'distinct from other occupations in that it has been given the right to control its own work' (Freidson 1983). This gives emphasis to the value of socialising new entrants to nursing into the caring role through exposure to those elements which are said to be uniquely recognisable as nursing work. The reader is guided to the work of Melia (1987) for a detailed critique of this socialising process (see further reading section of Chapter 8).

Within the sociological literature 'professional' and 'professionalism' tend to attract writers from one of two main theoretical camps: (a) functionalism or (b) interactionist. You will have met these terms previously in Chapter 4 and they should be familiar. If not, please revise this section of the book before continuing. A functionalist view would, for example, describe a model of professionalism as beginning with a knowledge-based competence which is developed and held by experts (Rueschemeyer 1983). The competence is then accepted as pragmatically relevant for problems which are of importance to the client group as well as for others not immediately involved, such as immediate family. Rueschemeyer addresses the issue of social control as it applies to the functionalist model by suggesting that the recipients of expert services are not themselves adequately knowledgeable to solve their own problems or to assess the service themselves. She writes of the bargain struck with society to protect the population from incompetence, carelessness and exploitation. She goes on to say that professions regulate themselves, and the bargain is to exchange competence and integrity against the trust of the client and the wider community, relative freedom from 'non-expert' supervision and interference, protection against unqualified competition as well as a substantial remuneration and higher social status. There is a guarantee of regulation and self-control offered through stringent recruitment and training, formal organisation and informal relations among colleagues, codes of practice, high ethical standards and professional reinforcement of publicly stated codes through a professional standards' committee or, in appropriate cases, the courts.

Activity 9.1

1. Consider in some detail the notion of social control and the role played by health-care professionals in creating a dependency culture between them and their clients.

2. Obtain from your tutor an outline of the structure and function of the United Kingdom Central Council for Nursing, Midwifery and Health Visiting (UKCC). Study this carefully and make a judgement as to whether the functionalist model as described by Rueschemeyer applies to the organisation and running of the UKCC. If you think the model applies then list the reasons why.

An alternative to the functionalist view can be found in the writings of Atkinson (1983) who describes the approach taken by symbolic interactionists of the Chicago school. This school of thought reflects an unease about the very idea of 'profession' and 'professionalism' as a legitimate area for study, and that the search for a criterion-led definition is wrong. The Chicago school says that 'profession' should be construed in lay terms with no precise meaning attached to it. This means that occupations claim professional status under certain conditions and at particular times which, in other words, means 'when it suits them to do so'. In this sense it becomes a symbolic label which some occupational groups demand, and which may be granted by others. If we consider the history of nursing, it can be seen that branches such as mental health and learning disability nursing were always subordinate to general nursing, particularly at a time when virtually all care was offered on an institutional basis. The notion of either branch being afforded full nursing standing was spurious. The evolvement to full and equal status with their general nursing counterparts was not an easy road and many obstacles needed to be addressed and overcome. The main obstacles seemed to emanate from arrogance, elitism and failure to appreciate the problems of providing acceptable care to a client group that attracted the label 'Cinderella' and whose principal reason for being in care was not related to physical illness. Care was also provided in the unacceptable surroundings of long-stay institutions that were viewed as degrading and impersonal. There remained for many years a widely held view among general nurses that people who provided care for a 'mentally handicapped' or 'mentally ill' client group were themselves of inferior status. Even though the former General Nursing Councils maintained separate registers for mental illness and mental handicap nurses, this label of inferiority began to lessen only when the proposals within Project 2000 (UKCC 1985) became a reality. This represented a stage in the evolution of nursing education when, in the eyes of the Statutory Body for Nursing, Midwifery and Health Visiting, all branches of nursing were accorded equal importance and the terms 'mental illness' and 'mental handicap' were eventually changed to mental health and learning disabilities, respectively.

Even in the case described above where a powerful group (general nursing) bestowed equal rights to perceived inferior partners, symbolic interactionists would claim that:

> 'Despite the wealth of connotations attached to the title (*in this case Nurse*) there is nothing inherent in the work, training, values or whatever, which marks out the occupation so designated.'
> (Atkinson 1983:227) (Author's italics)

Of further relevance is the original work of Bucher & Strauss (1961) who say that an assumption of relative homogeneity within any profession is not entirely useful. They remark on the many identities, values and interests which permeate through professional or occupational groups. They use the term 'segments' when referring to different interests and outlooks within an occupation, and suggest that occupations strive not only to attain professional status and the maintenance of position, but that segments are also engaged in pressing their particular interests. Clearly, it can be seen that, in the struggle to attain full recognition within the nursing profession, the two groups described above took on a segmented role and relied on strong voices within their ranks to stake a claim over a lengthy period of time for equal status.

Reflection point 9.1

Consider carefully the symbolic interactionist point of view with respect to nursing. Try to reach a personal conclusion regarding nursing's claim for full professional status in the light of this point of view. The questions you should ask yourself are:

1. Is there anything in nursing that could be described as uniquely inherent to the work?
2. How did the label 'profession' come to be attached to nursing and who put it there?

Freidson (1983) offers the opinion that some definition of profession is essential if the concept of 'professionalisation' is to be understood. He says that it is not possible to study 'process' without a definition guiding one's focus, any more fruitfully than one can study 'structure' without a definition. Freidson identifies two major distinctions which can be applied to the concept of professionalisation. First, there is the broad sector of prestigious but varied occupations whose members have all had some measure of higher education and whose identification is more through educational status than their specific occupational skills. It has been commented that the move of nurse education into higher education would create a similar position whereby nursing falls into this category. Second, there are those occupations which demonstrate commonality of particular ideologies and institutional traits, which enable us to think of professionalism as a way of organising an occupation. Over and above the consideration of status, ideologies and traits can be refocused to bow to current market forces. It is noteworthy that most of the major theoretical writers on professions have all addressed themselves to professions in this second case (Freidson 1983).

Reflection point 9.2   Consider the extent to which nursing has changed to meet the resulting challenges both in primary and secondary care instigated by the internal market approach to managing the National Health Service.

A Crisis of Confidence

From the discussion so far it can be said that nursing represents a complex mixture of functionalism, symbolic interactionism and parochialism. There are powerful figures who pushed forward the claim for full professional status, such as Pyne (1981), Clay (1987) and more recently Kershaw (1995). Alternatively, one of the original sociological thinkers (Etzioni 1969) aligned nursing to the minor professions. Such a view may still exist within the current management ethos of the Health Service which is evidenced by the decline in nursing power at the higher management level.

It is worth mentioning that the late Trevor Clay was the General Secretary of the Royal College of Nursing (RCN) at the time of the Report of the Commission on Nursing Education chaired by Dr Harry Judge (RCN 1985) (The Judge Report). The RCN Council instigated this commission on the grounds of impatience with the pace of gradualism from a system dominated by service-led educational policy to one which placed the education of nurses firmly within the Higher Education sector. Clay defended any possible charge of academic elitism by maintaining that student nurses would not be removed from their traditional places of clinical experience, namely hospital wards and community care settings. This maintained the identification of nursing as being essentially practice focused with the difference being that students would be supernumerary to staffing requirements. Clearly, nursing education has undergone considerable change in a relatively short time. This change grew from an earlier crisis of confidence in the education of nurses throughout the United Kingdom where curricular content and methods of delivery were placed firmly under the spotlight.

Schon (1987) implies that, where there is a crisis of confidence in professional education, there exists a corresponding crisis in professional knowledge.

> 'If professions are blamed for ineffectiveness and impropriety, their schools are blamed for failing to teach the rudiments of effective and ethical practice.'
> (Schon 1987:8)

One of the main tenets supporting the right to be called a profession is that a strong evidence-based element exists which in turn yields knowledge applicable to everyday practice (Schein 1973). When seen through Freidson's eyes this represents an attempt to bring the two major distinctions of prestige and commonality together in providing a practitioner whose preparation for practice stems from a high-status educational system whilst retaining specific occupational skills linked by research evidence.

Trade Unions and Professional Associations

In a traditional sense the label **profession** applies only to a select group of occupations such as medicine, law and the priesthood. Earlier we discussed the twin elements of distinctiveness and control which mark out a profession from other 'lower status' occupational groups, resulting in professions such as medicine developing elitist and impregnable structures that govern, regulate and protect well-established vocational ideologies. Powerful professional bodies such as the Royal Colleges represent the different factions of medicine and will quite readily take on central government should these ideologies be threatened in any way. The British Medical Association (BMA) has a long history of opposing Government reforms where threats to vested interests are perceived and, in some ways, acts as a Trade Union for its members. Despite internal differences and tensions within the Royal Colleges and the BMA, doctors can always be relied on to display unity in the face of serious political attempts to reorganise them. Unlike nursing, medicine will not allow itself to be split or weakened in any way and, as Hart (1996) points out, 'The divisions between nursing's trade unions and professional associations is almost unique in labour history indicating nursing's position somewhere between a skilled trade and a profession' (Hart

1996:5). Historically, the marked ideological differences separating the Royal College of Nursing (RCN) from Health Service Trade Unions such as the Confederation of Health Service Employees (COHSE) were damaging to unity. Hart (1996) says that these differences were deeply significant, nowhere more so than when industrial action was being considered. Until recently, the RCN remained totally opposed to its members taking any form of industrial action on the grounds that patients and clients would suffer. This position also confirmed the RCN as being an organisation 'uniquely promoting the advance of nursing as a profession and the professional standing and interests of its members' (Hart 1996:9).

COHSE has since merged with the National Union of Public Employees (NUPE) and the National Association of Local Government Officers (NALGO) to form Unison, the country's largest trade union. The Royal College of Nursing has changed its stance on industrial action and will now permit its members to take limited action in pursuit of employment grievances. Common ground does exist between these organisations but historical differences still prevail and it could be said that the bargaining power of nursing is weakened as a result.

Reflection point 9.3

The argument against nurses taking strike action is that it would harm patients and clients as well as demeaning the high regard that the general public have for nursing.

Where do you stand on this issue? Could such action ever be justified?

Vocationalism v Professionalism

The arguments surrounding professionalism and vocationalism have plagued nursing for many years. In attempting to unravel the complexities of these terms it is necessary to visit the early history of nursing and consider the powerful and enduring influences that guided early nurses, thus laying a foundation from which the modern service could evolve. Nursing has its roots in a notion of vocationalism that puts the sick, handicapped and vulnerable person at the very heart of the caring role. It is a selfless, dedicated role that pays little heed to personal remuneration, requiring the carer to work long hours without complaint and often putting her or his own health at risk. Nursing, evolving as it does from holy orders, reflects the rigid discipline and dedication to duty that was expected of people in such orders. The title 'sister' clearly originates from this early period in history and the matrons reflected a role that could be construed as once being occupied by the Mother Superior. There is an emphasis placed on status whereby a junior nurse could be equated with the novice entering a convent to test out her vocation. Junior nurses similarly tested out their suitability for the work by undertaking the menial tasks and being subjected to a harsh disciplinary regime. There is also a military influence in the way that nursing organised itself into distinct levels of rank. For example, there were special areas such as dining rooms and sitting rooms set aside for those of higher rank. Matrons had the luxury of being waited on hand and foot by personal maids, and senior sisters could expect a high level of service in their personal dining areas. Uniforms and insignia reflect the military influence which to some extent still remains; indeed, in my early years as a student we had to parade each morning in uniform to be inspected by the principal tutor before formal classes began. Another expectation was that floors would be polished to a high degree through manual means and the Principal's desk would receive similar attention. Penalties existed to punish the whole group for any fall in the standard of one member.

Let us refer back to the quotation by Warr in which it is suggested that vocationalism is inextricably linked to practical day-to-day nursing work and the performance of all the jobs required by the patient or client, no matter how mundane. He says that the true nature of nursing can be revealed by taking a reflective view, using the vocational ideology as the vehicle through which this reflection can occur. He argues that much of the debate surrounding the professionalisation of nursing centres on the 'unique nature' of its knowledge base and related practice. In defending this somewhat rigid stance it could be argued that nursing has built barriers against the recognition of vocational awards which it views as substandard, particularly in respect of assessment criteria and care outcomes (Le Var 1996). The early ideology of 'vocation', derived from a pragmatic philosophy of caring at the very centre of nursing, seems to have been abandoned in the pursuit of professionalism. There is a view that vocational work is less demanding than professional work, carried out by people with lesser or no formal qualifications.

However, Jarvis (1997) does not make this distinction and, by taking the stance that 'vocational education refers to every occupation' (Jarvis 1997:26), he strongly refutes professional elitism. He quotes primary sources (Kerr et al 1973) in support of the thesis that occupational educational systems do not primarily exist to conserve traditional values. The marketplace will dictate what goes into the curriculum and Jarvis maintains that as a result of the global information explosion we must realign how we think about our own occupation. He suggests that a massive growth in continuing vocational education has become pre-eminent and will continue into the forseeable future, guided to a large extent by employers who will define training and educational needs based on budgetary restrictions, new caring philosophies and European legislation.

Reflection point 9.4

> By taking a clear stand in support of nursing qualifications and their superiority to vocational awards it could be argued that nursing is short-sighted and is creating a policy that will provide opportunities for health trusts to cut costs by employing more vocational carers and fewer professional nurses.
>
> In your opinion, where does nursing currently stand regarding its status in the marketplace of caring?

The Generalist Nurse

We can now move on to consider another contentious issue: that of the generalist nurse. Recent literature (Barr & Sines 1996) reminds us of the substantial differences that exist between preregistration nurse education in the UK and many of our European partners. These authors point out that for nursing in the majority of other European countries discrete educational branches do not exist and that the system operated in the UK is viewed, by some (but not all), as an expensive luxury. Under current conditions a section of the UK nurse population who qualify in certain specialist branches of care would not be elible for employment in other countries within Europe because their specialism is not recognised.

Arguments For Generalism

It is argued that a move towards a generalist approach would greatly enhance employment opportunities on mainland Europe particularly if there were an agreement between the training authorities for standard preregistration preparation. In support of the generalist nurse Barr & Sines (1996) do not suggest a cessation of specialist preparation but recognise that opportunities for postregistration development could follow logically from a broad initial generalist preparation. This seems to fit quite well with the arguments discussed earlier where Jarvis (1997) makes the case for greater emphasis to be placed on continuing vocational education. If a generalist course of academic study and related practice becomes the norm for nursing in the UK then we may see the philosophy behind the present Common Foundation Programme extended across three years, giving greater emphasis to the notion of commonality. Ensuing postgeneralist preparation would provide nursing with a truly specialist set of pathways which it is argued we do not have at present.

A proposal by the Royal College of Nursing (1997) suggests a number of principles that would provide a new foundation for future education and training. The RCN seems to favour a generalist approach to the first three years leading to a Bachelor degree in nursing where students would graduate in a chosen field of care but have a sound background in all aspects of basic nursing practice and theory. Then a postgraduate specialist year would become available leading to honours in one of a number of specialisms including adult nursing, learning disability and mental health nursing, palliative care and caring for the older person. The proposal also called for a widening of the entry gate to facilitate applicants from a number of different routes, including level 3 SVQ/NVQ or level 3 GSVQ/GNVQ. The RCN also proposed a different kind of one year foundation programme that could be delivered by Colleges of Further Education that collaborate with local higher education providers of nursing programmes.

Arguments Against Generalism

A section of the UK nursing fraternity has expressed concerns that a move towards generalism would result in a dilution of skills held and practised by nurses particularly in those areas that attract the title 'specialist'. These areas would include mental health, learning disability and children's nursing. There is an existing perception held by many mental health nurses that the Diploma in Higher Education (UKCC 1985) has always militated against their speciality and put forward powerful arguments to support increased specialism rather than the reverse. It is suggested by opponents to generalism that to rely only on generalist preparation would produce practitioners that were less clinically skilled than at present, with a consequence that standards of care would suffer. Health service managers may find the proposals for generalism financially attractive because the need to commit expensive resourses to specialist training and supervision in the clinical areas would cease. Generalism would in effect create a position not dissimilar to that described earlier in the chapter in which the hierarchy of nursing would be dominated by a general emphasis to care with the specialisms subverted to a subordinate role. There are strong arguments to suggest that a move towards generalism would create disunity in the nursing ranks. For example, Barr & Sines (1996) are of the opinion that advances made in the nursing care of people with learning disabilities and those with mental health problems would be lost if future legislation took account of the fact that many European countries do not recognise these branches of nursing. Without a vigorous postregistration programme, provision for nursing in these and other specialist fields would be noticeably reduced or eliminated completely. The arguments surrounding postregistration education in the specialist fields of nursing are taken further in the next section.

Reflection point 9.5

Having read some of the advantages and disadvantages of generalism offered by others, reflect on your own views. Ask yourself the following questions:

1. Would generalism be attractive to health service managers because it provides opportunities for cutting costs?
2. In the face of generalism are concerns expressed about skill dilution real and well founded?
3. Would a growth in commonality set back progress in the care of vulnerable groups that do not naturally fall into generalist categories?

The Decline of Institutional Care and Changes in Hospital Provision

Health care delivery is a constant feature of the political agenda. Each of the mainstream political parties in the UK have a vested interest in maintaining a form of national health service; therefore, whichever party holds the balance of power there will be a policy on health that addresses this issue. In the past decade we have witnessed major changes in patterns of care delivery. Perhaps the most far reaching change has been the rapid decline in institutional care for people with mental health problems and those with learning disablies. The Victorian philosophies of care which included the use of large impersonal and often isolated mental institutions for housing and treating people with these kinds of problems and disabilities have finally given way to more civilised methods of health-care delivery. These institutions have gone the way of the other well-known Victorian edifice to a caring society – the workhouse.

Primary health care is now an established feature of caring for this and other sections of society that require specific treatment. Alongside these changes in mental health provision we have witnessed changes in the general provision of health care. For example, as part of the drive for efficiency the Conservative government in the 1990s pledged a reduction in waiting times for surgical operations. As a consequence there has been a growth in popularity for day hospitals that provide non-urgent surgical services. Such a policy moves the onus for postoperative care from the hospital to the general practitioner and/or the community nursing service. In many cases, because of early discharge, more responsibility for care is transferred to the family and in some cases directly to the service user. A phenomenon of modern health care has been the rapid growth in the numbers of informal carers who by definition are untrained and unpaid, thereby saving the government huge amounts of money that hitherto would have been spent on in-hospital provision. A more detailed discussion on the role of informal caring is provided in Chapter 11 but at this point you are asked to consider the following case study.

Case study 9.1

Allan is a 50-year-old man who is classified as being severely learning disabled. He lives with his elderly widowed mother in warden-controlled accommodation. His mother is not in the best of health but has a strong wish to continue caring for him for as long as possible. Allan receives regular visits from the community learning disability nurse and a carer visits the home to carry out basic housekeeping tasks. His mother receives care from the general practitioner and is seen by the district nurse who regularly calls to change dressings on an ulcerated leg.

This scenario is not uncommon. In many cases such as the one described here it is only a matter of time before the carer reaches a point at which it is not possible to carry on, and alternative provision has to be considered. The ideal situation is for service providers to be involved in promoting a supportive relationship with informal carers and there is evidence of this happening already within the context of community mental health and learning disability nursing (Parrish & Birchenall 1997). Parrish & Birchenall (1997) use as an example the initiatives contained within a document entitled 'Continuing the Commitment' (DoH 1995) which identifies the changing role of the learning disability nurse in the face of changing health-care practices within the National Health Service. From a day-to-day work perspective, boundary crossing is central to the future effectiveness of this branch of nursing, particularly as the nurse becomes more skilled in specialist areas such as health education, health surveillance, dietetics, as well as the more general issues associated with physical, social and psychological care. Even with the possible advent of the generalist nurse the arguments for the retention of a specialist practitioner in this area of care are strongly supported within this document.

Parrish & Birchenall write:

'How nurses, managers and other primary healthcare workers manage change will have a major effect on future service development and the quality of life of the individuals using these services. The resulting swing towards primary healthcare set around general practice and primary healthcare teams provides a powerful opportunity for nurses who care for people with learning disability to become key players in shaping the services of their clients. . . . Through teamwork, it is possible to provide a more effective service for people with learning disabilities.'

(Parrish & Birchenall 1997:92)

<table>
<tr><td>Reflection
point 9.6</td><td>Arguments against dispensing with the services of psychiatric hospitals suggest that the loss of an 'asylum' environment in which vulnerable people were supposedly cushioned and protected against intolerance and prejudice places them and society in jeopardy.

In the light of the closure of these hospitals carefully consider the quote by Parrish and Birchenall and reflect on your own views of how vulnerable people should be cared for.</td></tr>
</table>

Normalisation

The term **normalisation** gained initial prominence when it appeared in the Danish Mental Retardation Act of 1959. From this time the theories and application of normalisation remain central to the provision of human services for a cross section of vulnerable and devalued people in society. It provides the main direction for the movement towards 'an ordinary life' for citizens who in some way find themselves disenfranchised from mainstream society. Normalisation owes its popularity to the seminal work of Nirje (1969), Wolfensberger (1972) and Bank-Mikkelson (1980). Further work carried out by Wolfensberger in 1983 describes the notion of 'social role valorisation', thus adding credence to the underpinning philosophy of normalisation as being strongly associated with the creation of valued social roles for hitherto stigmatised groups.

Normalisation as a concept has often been misunderstood. It is not about making people 'normal' in the sense of them being originally abnormal and then magically restored to normal functioning. It is about understanding a shared set of values and beliefs that form the fabric of a civilised society and enabling people to fit in and feel comfortable in their social role. It is a useful exercise to compare the respective definitions of normalisation as described by Nirje, Wolfensberger and Bank-Mikkelson (Definitions box 9.1).

Of the three principal authors mentioned it is Wolfensberger who is the most quoted in nursing literature. He has gained wide-ranging respect and his work continues to influence multiprofessional education. His theories provide a number of important areas for boundary crossing, thus making it possible for formal and informal carers to work together in a climate of trust and understanding.

We have seen that the early theories supporting normalisation centre on the 'hidden' stigmatised groups who received care in the closed environments of long-stay hospitals. However, the concept of normalisation is moving towards a broader base; for example primary health-care teams refer to the normalisation of the 'sick' child. Many children, who suffer renal problems and traditionally experienced long-term care in the clinical environment of the hospital are now living at home where

Definitions box 9.1	Definitions of normalisation
	Nirje 'Making available to mentally retarded people patterns of life and conditions as close as possible to the regular circumstances and ways of life of society.' (Nirje 1969)
	Wolfensberger 'Utilization of means which are as culturally normative as possible, in order to establish and/or maintain personal behaviours and characteristics which are as culturally normative as possible.' (Wolfensberger 1972)
	Bank-Mikkelson 'Making normal mentally retarded people's housing, education, working and leisure conditions. It means bringing them the legal and human rights of all other citizens.' (Bank-Mikkelson 1980)

their medical and care needs are provided in a normal familiar environment. The child in this case is no longer isolated and by re-joining the community maintains a social role simply by becoming visible.

Reflection point 9.7	Consider other examples of how the general principles of normalisation and social role valorisation can be be used to improve the quality of life for other vulnerable groups. For example, older people placed in care who suffer some form of dementia may well become 'hidden' from society by virtue of their condition.

Professions Allied to Medicine

Occupations that fall into the category of Professions Allied to Medicine (PAMs) include physiotherapy, occupational therapy, radiography, speech therapy, audiology and cardiology. The educational and professional infrastructure related to these professions is firmly established and they each have a highly specialist body of knowledge from which practice is drawn. In this sense they are not dissimilar to nursing which has for many years attempted to define a body of knowledge unique to itself that can be applied whatever specialism is being practised. As seen earlier in this chapter the label of elitism can easily be attached to occupational groups that make claims for unique knowledge and status; they become isolated from other groups working in the same care environment and negative rivalries soon develop. It is on this basis that the notion of shared learning has developed in popularity, with the crossing of educational and practice boundaries being high on the training agenda. A government White Paper 'The NHS:

a service with ambitions' (DoH 1996) showed a political will to create a climate for sharing and placed emphasis on the need for multiprofessional and effective team working. The White Paper also gave support to the continued development of existing partnerships in education. Recent initiatives in this area include the setting up by the Department for Education and Employment (DfEE) in 1996 of a series of occupational networks including one that is dedicated to the dissemination of flexible learning developments in the field of health-care education. A network such as this creates a positive sharing climate within which people can exchange ideas with the ultimate goal of improving services. Once the barriers of suspicion are removed and cross-professional dialogue begins it is surprising just how much in common each group has with one another. Claims to unique knowledge become more difficult to justify when it is found that whole subject areas are shared; good examples are communication skills, health promotion, disability studies, research and human physiology.

According to Friend (1997) some of the best examples of shared learning are to be found in accident and emergency departments where the emphasis on training is problem-focused.

> 'Where the whole of the team goes on, say, a paediatric trauma course, and it doesn't matter whether you are a nurse or a doctor, you can participate because it is such a specialist area. You have got a reason to be there because it is directly related to patient outcome.'
> (Friend 1997:20)

The same author presents a case study of shared learning in which it is suggested that the logistics are difficult but the benefits are many. The health service is certainly moving towards multi-skilling and, as Friend says, 'this involves a sort of coming together of the professions'. It is also proposed in this case study:

> 'that if newly qualified professionals are to participate in "some sort of interprofessional enterprise", then exposure to and experience of this during their professional education will make them more attractive to prospective employers.'
> (Friend 1997:20)

Reflection point 9.8

Reflect on the knowledge you already have about nursing.

Have you experienced shared learning with students from other health-care professions? If so, identify those areas where the process of sharing provided insight into the wider perspectives of health care.

If you have not experienced shared learning could you identify any benefits that may accrue from doing so?

Market Forces in a Changing Economy of Care

The power of market forces on the employability of nurses is quite profound. The mixed economy of care which embraces the public, private and voluntary sectors has produced a spectrum of caring that places nurses in an invidious position. They are now quite likely to be competing for posts with lesser qualified and cheaper-to-employ people. For example, this can be seen quite clearly in the area of learning disabilities. Nurses whose training and experience was largely confined to the institutional model of care experienced great difficulty when caring provision was transfered to the community and the social model replaced the medical model. Specialist nursing competencies became redundant and regrettably so did many of the nurses. New forms of care demand new capabilities and nurses in this field had to adapt or risk being completely submerged under an overwhelming tide of change. Lower level social-work qualifications were valued more highly than nursing qualifications and those nurses who gained employment often found themselves in subordinate positions to lesser qualified and inexperienced managers. Leaving the relative security of institutional care for the unknown world of multi-agency working in the community plunged nursing into situations where different value bases, occupational histories, professional boundary demarcation and jealously-guarded professional relationships dramatically affected the working environment. Nursing became a small fish in a large pool and survival meant adjusting to new situations and tensions often ran high. More recently there has been a move towards greater recognition of the value of nursing within the multi-agency environment. This may well be a reflection on improved educational standards that now exist in nursing education and also the ability of nurses to change with the times.

The growth in the private residential nursing-home sector for elderly people has also created a situation in which much of the care is provided by care assistants with or without minimal National Vocational Qualifications supervised by a small number of registered nurses. It is not a requirement for these registered nurses to hold a recognised specialist qualification in care of elderly people, although a number of them do. Economics is the main driving force behind the provision of care in the three sectors previously described. The balance sheet determines the level of care that can be offered, and staffing profiles often reflect the economic position of the organisation in question, whether it be a complex health trust or a small nursing home. The Labour government elected in 1997 pledged in its manifesto to ensure a properly funded health service and to remove the inequalities created by the internal market. The effects of this should enable general practitioners to treat or refer patients according to need, not whether the treatment can be afforded.

**Activity
9.2**

Revise what is meant by the internal market of care and discover the origin of this controversial method of managing the health service.

Specialist Practice

The 1990s have witnessed a major change in direction for nurses that has taken them down the road towards specialist practice in an increasing number of areas. For example, there are now specialist courses in accident and emergency nursing, stoma care, challenging behaviour, psychotherapy, renal nursing, neonatal care and many others. You will recall that earlier in this chapter we discussed the advantages and disadvantages of generalism which included the notion of a broader foundation than at present with subsequent postregistration specialist preparation. It would seem that, with the proliferation of approved postregistration courses in a wide variety of specialist areas, there is a clear indication of the direction in which nursing is heading. The arguments for or against generalism and multiskilling may be worth revisiting, particularly as nursing has seemingly decided where it wants to be in respect of continuing professional development. Discussion has taken place on the various merits of specialist and advanced practice which led in 1996 to the UKCC conducting a listening exercise. This process of listening enabled members of the profession to have a say on what changes, if any, they wanted to see in respect of advanced and specialist practice.

It would seem that a clear consensus emerged from this exercise and a conclusion about the meaning of advanced practice became clear. The UKCC said in its Spring 1997 newsletter:

'It was felt that there are neither agreed definitions of advanced practice nor criteria against which standards for advanced practice can be set. It was also clear that most nurse practitioner graduates fill the requirements of specialist, rather than advanced, practice. For these reasons, it was felt that the UKCC, while fully supporting the notion of advanced practice, should avoid setting explicit standards but should consider how specialist practice could embrace nurse practitioners and clinical nurse specialists.'
(UKCC 1997:5)

From this it can be seen that the UKCC is unhappy about labelling any activity as advanced; instead, the council wishes for specialist practice to embrace as many practitioners as possible rather than be seen to support a policy of exclusiveness.

Each of the four main branches of nursing have major components that lend themselves to specialist practice, and a continuation of the existing policy of research will provide a substantial evidence base to support this assertion.

Summary   This chapter has ranged over a number of important issues relating to the professional status of nursing. We have discussed the notion of professionalism and examined some of the key elements relating to this. Having done so it is still unclear whether nursing is a profession or not; it largely depends on which definition is used. What does seem to be clear, however, is the necessity for nursing regularly to change direction, continually to re-examine its educational and practice infrastructure, and to cross occupational boundaries.

Further Reading

Elston MA 1991 The politics of professional power: medicine in a changing service. In: Cabe J, Calnan M, Bury M (eds) The sociology of the health service. Routledge, London
    This chapter provides further insight into professional autonomy in the exercise of legitimate control and authority over professional activity.

Hart C 1994 Behind the mask: nurses, their trade unions and nursing policy. Baillière Tindall, London
    This book charts the historical development of health service trade unions and their counterparts, the professional organisations. Hart analyses their present day contribution to modern health care and the development of nursing policy, and provides fascinating commentary on the similarities and differences within the respective roles and functions of trade unions and professional organisations operating within the National Health Service.

References

Atkinson P 1983 The reproduction of the professional community. In: Dingwall R, Lewis P (eds) The sociology of the professions. Macmillan, London
Bank-Mikkelson 1980 Denmark. In: Flynn RJ, Nitsch KE (eds) Normalisation, social integration and community services. Pro-Ed, Austin, Texas
Barr O, Sines D 1996 The development of the generalist nurse within pre-registration nurse education in the UK: some points for consideration. Nurse Education Today 16(4): 274–277
Birchenall M, Baldwin S, Morris J 1997 Learning disability and the social context of caring. (Healthcare Active Learning.) Open Learning Foundation/Churchill Livingstone, Edinburgh
Bucher R, Strauss AL 1961 Professions in process. American Journal of Sociology 60: 325–334
Clay T 1987 Nurses: power and politics. Heinemann, London

Department of Health (DoH) 1995 Continuing the commitment: the report of the learning disability project. DoH, London

Department of Health (DoH) 1996 The NHS: a service with ambitions. White Paper, DoH, London

Etzioni A (ed) 1969 The semi professions and their organisation. Free Press, New York

Freidson E 1983 The theory of professions: state of the art. In: Dingwall R, Lewis P (eds) The sociology of the professions. Macmillan, London

Friend B 1997 Two heads. The Health Services Journal 6, March: 19–20

Hart C 1996 The great divide. International History of Nursing Journal 1(3): 5–17

Jarvis P 1997 The globalisation of nurse education within higher education. Nurse Education Today 17(1): 22–30

Kerr C, Dunlop G, Harbison F, Myers C 1973 Industrialism and industrial man, 2nd edn. Penguin, Harmondsworth

Kershaw B 1995 Active thinkers. Nurse Education Today 15(3): 159–160

King I 1981 A theory for nursing: systems, concepts, process. Wiley, New York

Le Var RMH 1996 NVQs in nursing, midwifery and health visiting: a question of assessment and learning? Nurse Education Today 16(2): 85–93

Melia K 1987 Learning and working: the occupational socialisation of nurses. Tavistock, London

Nirje B 1969 The normalisation principle and its human management implications. In: Kugel RB, Wolfensberger W (eds) President's Committee on Mental Retardation. Changing patterns in residential services for the mentally retarded. Retardation, Washington DC

Parrish A, Birchenall P 1997 Learning disability nursing and primary healthcare. British Journal of Nursing 6(2): 92–98

Pyne RH 1981 Professional discipline in nursing: theory and practice. Blackwell, London

Royal College of Nursing (RCN) 1985 The education of nurses: a new dispensation – Commission on nurse education. (The Judge Report.) RCN, London

Royal College of Nursing (RCN) 1997 Shaping the future of nursing education: a discussion document. RCN, London

Rueschemeyer D 1983 Professional autonomy and the social control of expertise. In: Dingwall R, Lewis P (eds) The sociology of the professions. Macmillan, London

Schein E 1973 Professional education. McGraw Hill, New York

Schon DA 1987 Educating the reflective practitioner: towards a new design for teaching and learning in the professions. Jossey Bass, San Francisco

United Kingdom Central Council for Nursing, Midwifery and Health Visiting (UKCC) 1985 Project 2000: a new preparation for practice. UKCC, London

United Kingdom Central Council for Nursing, Midwifery and Health Visiting (UKCC) 1997 Register, Spring. UKCC, London

Warr JG 1996 Vocationalism: a mirror on the profession. Nurse Education Today 16(4): 267–269

Wolfensberger W 1972 The principle of normalization in human services. National Institute on Mental Retardation, Toronto

Wolfensberger W 1983 Social role valorization: a proposed new term for the principle of normalization. Mental Retardation 21: 234–239

HEALTH POLICY IN RELATION TO NURSING

Key concepts

- The NHS and Community Care Act 1990
- NHS Trusts
- GP contracts
- The Health of the Nation
- The founding of the NHS
- NHS reorganisation
- Purchaser/provider interactions
- Privatisation
- Cinderella services
- Community
- Informal care
- Informal carers
- Women as carers

In Section 4 the scene moves from nursing work to the wider arenas of the politics of health care. This section concentrates on the changing shape of the National Health Service (NHS). The National Health Service and Community Care Act (1990) is reviewed and discussed, with some emphasis on the impact of changes such as the inception of the internal market and Trust status.

Section 4 outlines and reviews that part of the 1990 NHS and Community Care Act which focuses on community care, and considers the possible reasons for emphasis on 'community' occurring at this time. This section is concerned with the social changes which have pre-empted these moves in the health-care system and the interpretations of the impact of such major changes on professional and client worlds.

Consideration is given to the 1997 Government White Paper on health entitled 'The New NHS. Modern. Dependable.' and particularly those proposals for change directed at the internal market and GP fundholding. The NHS is a dynamic institution and as such will continue to provide the nursing profession with challenges and opportunities for professional development. Section 4 provides historical and modern perspectives, giving food for thought as to the direction of Government policy and identifying possible avenues for nurses to explore.

10 The Changing Shape of the National Health Service

John Clayton

Key concepts
- The structure of the NHS in 1948
- A brief history of the reorganisations of the NHS
- The effect on health service provision of the NHS Act of 1990
- NHS trusts
- GP contracts
- Significant changes in health-care provision: provider/purchaser interactions and the 'mixed economy of care'
- The health of the nation
- Future predictions: changes with a Labour government

The National Health Service (NHS) has provided 'free' health care for the population of the UK for almost half a century. During that time the cost of the service has risen dramatically and consecutive governments have attempted to control this rise in expenditure by a series of reorganisations and structural changes. This chapter will examine these changes and analyse the success (or lack of success) of these initiatives.

Health Care Before the NHS

Before the establishment of the NHS in 1948, the majority of people living in Great Britain were not entitled to free medical care and treatment. The 1911 'Health Insurance Act' had introduced medical insurance aimed at providing general practitioner (GP) services for working people (hospital services were not included). The dependants of the workers were not 'covered' by this scheme. Working people paid medical insurance payments to 'Friendly Societies' and in return received medical care and family support during times of their illness and inability to work. The healthy worker was expected to pay for the health care needs of his family if they became ill (Moore 1993:93).

This inequality in provision of health care had long been criticised in the interwar years (1919–1939) by a number of important sources. The 'Dawson' report of 1920, for example, highlighted the need to extend the maintenance of health, stating that 'curing of disease should be made available to all citizens' and the British Medical Association (BMA) in 1930 advocated extending the existing medical insurance schemes to cover the dependants of working people.

This inequality in health care was not only limited to primary care. Within the hospital sector receipt of services often depended on the ability of the individual to pay for treatment. Even the Voluntary hospitals, traditionally introduced to meet the needs of the poor, were unable to extract sufficient funds from charitable donations during the 1930s and were forced to attract payment from private patients to ensure their survival. (In a limited way this could be seen as a **mixed economy of care**, a model which was to find governmental favour in the 1990s.)

At the outbreak of the Second World War, these inequalities were forced to the forefront of the political agenda as the government, fearful of civilian casualties from enemy bombing raids as well as injured service men and women, took overall charge of the nation's hospitals and introduced the Emergency Medical Service. The observed deficiency in hospital facilities led to a growing consensus throughout the wartime years that the UK was in need of a National Health Service, comprehensive and free to all citizens. Health was part of the collectivist ideology of social welfare of the time, an ideology which encompassed social services, housing, employment and social security as well as education, and was symbolised in the Beveridge report of 1942, of which the stated intent was that of government intervention to tackle the 'five giants' – disease, ignorance, squalor, idleness and want.

Thus, during the course of the Second World War there was a general, broad and growing agreement of politicians, health professionals and the citizens of the UK that there was a public need for a National Health Service, free for all and designed to tackle the existing inequalities in health-care provision. This mood can be identified in the article by Dr Maurice Newfield, entitled 'A real medical service', which appeared in *Picture Post* on 4 January 1941.

'What we want are:

- A State Medical Service
- The full benefit of medical science available to everybody
- A health centre for every district

In this matter of individual and social health our aims are as revolutionary as they are simple and attainable. First and foremost is the greatest health of the greatest number. Definitely second in importance is the cure of diseases we fail to prevent and the alleviation of those we fail to cure.... We must do everything possible not only to advance knowledge of the diagnosis, prevention and treatment of disease, but to ensure that facilities for the application of this knowledge are available for every man, woman and child in the country.'

(Newfield 1941:36)

Activity 10.1   Interview a person who is old enough to remember the provision of health services before the NHS was established. How were health services delivered to individual people, and how did people pay for their health care? Put yourself in the shoes of someone who had to pay or barter for health care. Is this an acceptable way of obtaining essential care?

The aims were certainly revolutionary and, though eventually attainable, the process of attainment was anything but simple. Moreover, the blend of prevention and treatment that Newfield identified has never been totally satisfied, as the NHS has tended to focus on curing the sick whereas the prevention of ill health has traditionally been the subordinate partner.

Despite the growing wealth of opinion and agreement in the need for a national health service, there was still a great deal of political debate and argument before the service was established. Most of the disagreements centred around the individual interests of the specific players, the politicians and the medical profession and to a lesser extent the local authorities.

As Klein observes 'Accepting a general notion is one thing, devising and implementing a specific plan is a very different matter' (Klein 1983:7).

The bitter exchanges and arguments which preceded the introduction of the NHS in 1948 largely demanded that Aneurin Bevan, the Minister for Health in the Labour government of 1946–1951, make a series of compromises to the members of the medical profession, recognising as he did that the service could not run without the commitment of the doctors. Bevan opted for a nationalisation of the hospital services rather than the extension of the insurance-based system of health care as advocated by the BMA. This service would give the government more central control, but the proposal ran the risk of offending the doctors. Bevan's concessions were that the teaching hospitals would be given special status, that consultants would be given a major role on the management of the service and that they would be able to retain private patients and offer them treatment using NHS facilities. In this way he acquired the support of the specialists and effectively split the medical profession. He did, however, offer the GPs certain concessions also to ensure their support for the service, by allowing them to retain their independent status and to receive their payments based on capitation fees, by the number of registered patients on their books. These agreements were not achieved without a great deal of bitter argument and counterargument. The power of the medical profession had been established and identified alongside other participants. In contrast, no concessions were made to the voluntary hospitals or any other health professionals including nurses, and the power of the local authorities in hospital management was greatly reduced. The successful negotiations of the medical profession in 1948 were probably a springboard for the disagreements and quarrels between politicians and doctors which were to infiltrate the future existence of the NHS. Flushed with the initial successes of these negotiations doctors could be excused for flexing their political muscle with future governments over a wide range of issues including resourcing, funding, government interference and, commonly, payment and working conditions.

And so the NHS was launched and the first seeds of medical technology were sown, seeds which would rapidly mature into a world of transplantations and keyhole surgery at phenomenal costs to successive governments. It is perhaps salient at this point to remember that this remarkable progress was made less than 100 years after the poorer citizens of Britain were often admitted to hospitals from which they were never discharged, whereas richer citizens paid privately for the right to be treated at home.

The NHS in 1948

The NHS came into existence on 5 July 1948. Funded largely by taxation it was effectively a tripartite structure, composed of three specific areas of health care with limited co-ordination or integration. The three areas of health care broadly covered:

- the hospital services
- the general practitioner services
- the local authority health and social services.

Supported by the assumption that the UK had a fixed quantity of ill-health, it was predicted that as the new service became universally available, the health of the population would gradually improve, thus reducing the need for the medical services and ultimately reducing the cost of the NHS bill. As successive governments became increasingly aware that the cost of the NHS was not going to fall, but on the contrary was likely to rise and carry on rising, there was a real incentive to control health service spending and to make the service more efficient and more accountable.

Changing Structures of the NHS: The Search for Efficiency and Control

The search for efficiency and financial control led to a reorganisation of the NHS in 1974. This reorganisation was intended to introduce a hierarchy of management from the government to local providers, which would allow the government greater financial and managerial control, while giving local providers the autonomy they needed to treat their clients. To this end 14 Regional Health Authorities (RHA) and 90 Area Health Authorities (AHA) were introduced. An attempt to tackle the problem of insufficient co-ordination between the various parts of the NHS was made by the introduction of positive links between the AHA and the local authorities, and the introduction of consensus management. The clients were also represented by the introduction of the Community Health Councils (CHC). These councils were introduced to safeguard the clients of the NHS and to assist them if there was a perceived reason for complaint. Unfortunately the councils were given no statutory powers to effect change in the health service and hence were only able to play a minor role in decision making. In other words, if a patient received a poor service and wished to complain, the CHC could advise the client how best to voice her or his complaint, the mechanism of the complaint and who to complain to, but was unable to become involved in the complaints procedure on the client's behalf. Similarly, although it was a legal right for CHCs to receive information about ward or hospital closures, they had no statutory powers to prevent this happening. For this reason the CHCs were often referred to as 'toothless watchdogs', and, although their role as an advisory and client help service is exemplary, their limited role in decision making has often been criticised.

The 1974 reorganisation was largely unsuccessful since it contributed to a period of industrial unrest, unlike anything witnessed before in the history of the NHS as doctors, nurses and other NHS employees became dissatisfied with their working conditions and low levels of pay and took industrial action. For example, in 1972 the ancillary workers went on strike in support of a £4.00 per week pay rise. The services were disrupted from October1972 into the spring of 1973 although the protesters eventually called off their strike without winning their claim. However, the industrial action was important since it disproved the belief that health service workers would never take strike action. Moreover, the number of health service workers who joined trade unions increased, and health unions began to employ leaders who were visibly more assertive, such as Rodney Bickerstaffe and Clive Jenkins. This increased assertiveness paid dividends and contributed to the successful series of pay settlements as Klein maintains: 'between 1970 and 1975, the average earnings of British workers rose by 107.8% whilst for ancillary workers the rise was 134% and for nurses 143%' (Klein 1983:112). Doctors were lagging behind and, so, unsurprisingly in 1975 junior hospital doctors took industrial action over pay and were successful in achieving increased payment for overtime work (above the 40 hours' basic week). There are two points are of interest here. First, the willingness of doctors to imitate other health service workers and take industrial action for the first time in their history and second the knock-on effect this had with consultants as the differential between registrars' salaries and consultants' salaries was eroded. The industrial action involving consultants centred around hospital pay beds, when the Labour government – as part of its manifesto commitment – tried to phase out pay beds in NHS hospitals. Pay beds allowed private patients to queue-jump and receive treatment earlier than NHS clients. The consultants reacted angrily to Labour's proposal, although the government received support from the TUC, which was antagonistic to pay beds and was aware that nurses and other health workers were being employed to treat these private patients before equally deserving NHS patients. When one considers the heated arguments that ensued, it is interesting to reflect what all the fuss was about since one's experience of health care in the 1980s and 1990s has led us to accept that queue-jumping by patients who can afford to pay has become common practice and furthermore has been openly encouraged by successive Conservative governments in the name of competition. The long, protracted and heated disagreements between the consultants and the Secretary of State for Health, Barbara Castle, forced the Prime Minister, Harold Wilson, to intervene and to invite Lord Goodman to act as a go-between. Although pay beds were separated from NHS provision in 1976, they were never completely phased out. Another major criticism of the reorganisation was that it was too mechanistic (Report of the Royal Commission on the NHS 1979) and that there were too many managerial tiers. One tier, the AHA, was removed in 1982 when a second major reorganisation of the NHS was implemented.

Activity 10.2   Look at Figure 10.1 part of which shows the structure of the NHS following the reorganisation of 1974. Compare it with Figure 10.2 which shows the structure of the NHS in 1996. List the main differences between the two structures.

The reorganisation of 1982 was a further attempt to increase efficiency and accountability. A total of 192 District Health Authorities

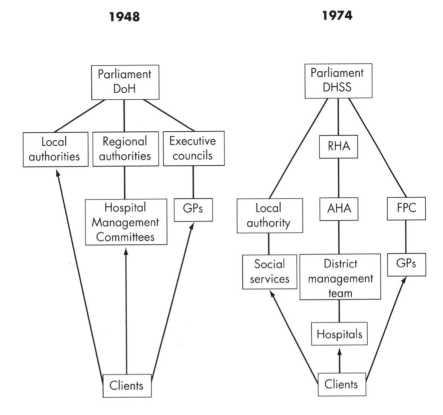

Figure 10.1 The structure of the NHS in 1948 and 1974

(DHAs) were introduced. Their role was as provider of services at the local level. They were given a far greater role in local decision making as the government followed a general policy of decentralisation. The DHAs also had links with the local authorities and with the CHCs. The task of the DHAs was made more difficult by the constraints on public spending which became a feature of the 1980s, and because the government still exerted formidable control on their planning capabilities. This led informed sources to question the relevance of the 1982 reorganisation (Alaszewski et al 1981).

The increased managerialism of the NHS evolved further in 1983 with the publication of the Griffiths report (Griffiths 1983). Although this report specified the importance of the client and the needs of client groups, it heralded the recruitment of general managers to the NHS and introduced a business model to health service delivery in direct contrast to the traditional health model which had persisted since 1948 (Allsop 1995).

The introduced business model met with bitter resentment by many practitioners within the NHS. Roy Griffiths had been the chairman of

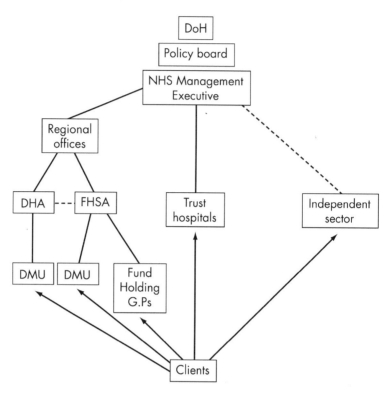

Figure 10.2 **The structure of the NHS in 1996**

Sainsburys plc and had been introduced into the health service to engender a business ethos, but health workers were suspicious of a manager with little or no knowledge of health care. Decisions in future would not be made on clinical good practice but on what could be afforded. This clash of cultures, introduced in 1983, was to remain with the NHS throughout the remaining years of Conservative government, a government which remained stubbornly preoccupied with the economic costs of the health service and with managerial responsibility and efficiency since Margaret Thatcher's (now Baroness Thatcher) first involvement, illustrated in the biographical comment:

> 'In significant ways, the NHS lacked the right economic signals to respond to these pressures. (The limitless demand for healthcare, free at the point of delivery and the demands of an increasing number of elderly people.) Dedicated though its staff generally were; cost conscious they were not.'
> (Thatcher 1993:607)

This preoccupation with economic issues has had a negative effect on staff morale within the NHS, and has resulted in feelings of indignation among practitioners that their working practices were wasteful and unconsidered. These feelings of vexation among health service practitioners were fuelled by the recognition that their critics did not possess the knowledge or skills to understand the detailed work involved, and the underlying discomfort at being forced to consider making a profit out of a person's ill-health fits uneasily with many health service workers.

Reflection point 10.1	Why do you think the government welcomed the findings of the Griffiths report (Griffiths 1983) and the recommendation that general managers should be recruited from the world of business rather than medicine?

Throughout the 1980s, the Conservative government under the premiership of Margaret Thatcher strived to increase the efficiency of the NHS and to develop professional accountability while constraining public spending. This led to the reforms of 1990 and the introduction of the 'NHS and Community Care Act', which were to have far-reaching effects for health and care services during the first half of the decade.

The NHS and Community Care Act 1990

A major change in British politics was signalled in 1979 with the election victory of the Conservative party with Margaret Thatcher at the helm. The new government had a large working majority, which gave it a powerful platform with which to introduce its policies. These policies were to have a direct influence on the NHS and included:

- more freedom for business
- more choice for clients
- removal of Trade Union influence in the Market
- reduced government interference in economic issues
    (Baggott 1994).

To increase choice in the NHS, the government offered people alternatives to the statutory services to which they had become accustomed (i.e. NHS and personal social services) and imposed on the citizens of Great Britain a mixed economy of health care. The growth of private medicine is a feature of the early years of the Thatcher administration, and clients were invited to choose their own health care and to pay accordingly. The resurgence of private health care was the very antithesis to the philosophy of the NHS with its statement of free health care for all. Moreover, with many people employed in low-wage professions, a recognised increase in part-time and temporary employment and with unemployment continuing to rise throughout the 1980s, the ability to pay for private health care was a privilege from which many of the citizens of the

UK were excluded. The Universalism of health care delivery, so important a factor in the establishment of the NHS, was consequently undermined and a two-tier system of health care, favouring the rich who could pay for services over the poor who could not, was encouraged.

For certain services, all the population (with the exception of citizens who were given exemptions, e.g. children) made their payments directly, as in, for example, prescription charges and eye tests. For other services, such as operations, clients who could afford it paid contributions to organisations providing health-insurance schemes. These organisations paid for the operations when their clients needed them. Employers, recognising the benefits of a healthy work force, began to offer health insurance to their employees as fringe benefits and were able to reap tax benefits. The government, supportive of private health care encouraged these changes hoping that a healthy private sector would alleviate the cost of the NHS bill. Many health service workers viewed the government's support for private health care as the death knell of the NHS and predicted that the success of the private sector would give the government the encouragement it needed to introduce an insurance-based NHS. Thatcher appears to dispute this point:

'Although I wanted to see a flourishing private sector of health alongside the National Health Service, I always regarded the NHS and its basic principles as a fixed point in our policies.'
(Thatcher 1993:606)

A basic principle of the NHS is that it should be a comprehensive service, free to all; this observation, however, is easy to argue against.

With the backing of employers and the government, more and more people became covered by private medical insurance as an alternative to the NHS, which was having difficulties with financial constraints. Clients were able to avoid waiting lists and had more control over their catering and accommodation requirements while they stayed in hospital, though it is unlikely that in many cases the standard of their health care was greatly improved. By 1986 25% of all hip replacement operations carried out in the UK were done privately (Nicholl et al 1989).

The influence of private health care in the local communities was equally important with the massive expansion of private residential homes and nursing homes, while the development of the voluntary and informal sectors contributed further to community provision. As in the area of health, however, these developments did not go uncriticised, and informed sources suggested that the sectors were a cheaper option and, once again, the likelihood that their expansion would lead to a two-tier system of health and social care was identified (see Chapter 11).

The expansion of the independent sector contributed to the problems

**Activity
10.3**

Find out if there is a private hospital in your locality (you could contact the CHC or Citizens Advice Bureau for this information). If your locality does have a private hospital, find out what services are provided and how much each specialty costs.

Points to consider include: the implication of differential ability to pay, and the range of services offered by private hospitals compared to the NHS.

experienced by the statutory sector, in particular the hospital service. In 1987 this resulted in a crisis, as recognised by the National Association of Health Authorities (NAHA 1987). Further support for these difficulties was proffered by the Royal Colleges (of Surgeons, Physicians, Obstetricians and Gynaecologists), who produced a joint statement highlighting the problems and requesting more funds. The service was close to breaking point, as Ham et al (1990) suggest, with temporary closures of wards and hospitals, and cancellations of operations. This forced the government to intervene, and despite speculation by health service workers that the government would replace taxation with social insurance as the funding model, the government elected to concentrate on a new initiative. This was the introduction of an internal market in which hospitals would compete with other hospitals and independent providers for services (Ham 1992).

**Reflection
point 10.2**

The 'hospital crisis' of 1987 forced the government to introduce new initiatives in health service management and provision, despite many people predicting a change in the funding mechanism, i.e. replace taxation by social insurance. Why do you think the government opted for an internal market of health services rather than a new funding model as the method of control?

The general management proposals of the 1983 Griffiths report were implemented as general managers were introduced at all levels of the NHS hierarchy. Many of these managers had little or no experience of health services but were co-opted from the world of business and the armed forces. These changes were explained in a government White Paper entitled 'Working for patients' (DoH 1989), which became the NHS Act in April 1990.

The major initiatives of the act were:

- the purchaser and provider role of the health service would be split
- the Department of Health would have two new boards: the NHS management executive and the policy board. These organisations would take overall control of management and policy issues respectively
- professional accountability would be increased.

The DHA became the major purchaser of secondary health care, a split from its role as provider. The role of provider was given to the hospitals which were invited to apply for Trust status. **Trust hospitals** are self-governing hospitals. They are run as individual businesses and unlike their predecessors must compete with other providers to obtain contracts from purchasers (Moore 1993:108). (See section on 'NHS Trusts' on p 209.)

The accountability of doctors was increased as general managers monitored their performance. The family practitioner committee (FPC) became the Family Health Services Authority (FHSA) and general managers were introduced into the management of the primary services, as the FHSA managed the contracts of the general practitioners, opticians, dentists and pharmacists within the community.

Case study 10.1

Jim is a 63-year-old ex-steel worker who took early retirement in order to spend more leisure time gardening and playing golf. However, these two hobbies became difficult for Jim to enjoy as he began to suffer from severe pains in his right hip. Jim visited his GP who suspected arthritis and referred him to the orthopaedic department of the local NHS Trust hospital. The consultant, Mr Hart, confirmed the diagnosis of arthritis and recommended that Jim underwent a hip replacement operation. The waiting time for the operation was approximately 9 months and Jim's name was added to the waiting list.

During the next month the pain in his hip got very much worse and Jim revisited his GP. His GP was a member of a fundholding practice and he recommended two alternative strategies. First, Jim was informed that he could 'go private', although, because he did not have any medical insurance, he would need to pay for the operation in full. The GP also suggested that it might be possible to get Jim an earlier operation in an NHS trust in another locality where the waiting time was shorter, providing Jim did not mind where the operation was performed. Jim decided to spend some of his redundancy money to hasten his hip replacement. He was surprised when 12 days later the consultant who performed the operation was Mr Hart. Two months after the operation Jim took out medical insurance for himself and his wife.

Jim is an example of a consumer of health services with a variety of providers. Notice that the DHA would have been the purchaser if Jim had elected to wait for his local NHS trust; the fundholding GP is the purchaser if an 'outside' trust is used by means of a 'cost per case contract' (these are relatively rare) or, as in this case, Jim is the purchaser if the private sector is used.

General practitioners with capitation of more than 9000 patients were invited to become fundholders with control of their own budgets and to purchase certain services from a variety of providers. General practitioners (whether fundholders or non-fundholders) remained the key providers of primary health care.

These changes encouraged a 'mixed economy of care' in which providers from the statutory sector, i.e. trusts, competed with other trusts, and with providers from the independent sector (private and voluntary) for client contracts.

A further development in the health of individuals was the change in emphasis from curative medicine to preventative health. This development continued in 1992 when a government White Paper entitled 'The Health of the Nation' (DoH 1992) was introduced, setting specific targets for a variety of preventable diseases such as cancer and heart disease.

NHS Trusts

In the new health structure trust hospitals became the main providers of hospital care. Other trusts became providers of community health services, and specialist providers, e.g. the ambulance service, were also encouraged to apply for trust status. The services provided by the trusts could be purchased by a range of purchasers, e.g. DHA, FHSA, fundholding GPs, etc. In April 1996 the DHA and the FHSA combined to become the major health service commissioning agency with a greatly increased purchasing capability. (See section on 'Significant changes in health care provision' on p 214 for more details on the effects of combined commissioning agencies on health service provision.) Trust hospitals were given self-governing status and, managed by a board of directors, were essentially individual businesses with autonomy to provide the services they felt were appropriate and to employ their own staff.

**Activity
10.4**   Visit your local hospital. Is the hospital a self-governing trust or a directly managed unit? What services does the hospital provide? Make a list of the services offered and compare these with the services provided by the private hospital you researched in Activity 10.3.

In 1990, during the first phase of trust applications, 66 hospitals applied for trust status of which 57 were approved. The second phase of 1992 realised a further 95 trusts, and 137 further trusts were approved in the third phase in 1993. Trust status confers upon the provider the ability to borrow money and to buy and sell property, though the trust must keep the public informed if it decides to sell property. This accountability is seen as a very important part of the NHS Act, and trust hospitals hold open meetings which members of the public are invited to attend, as well as publishing annual reports and keeping the CHC informed of changes in provision, such as ward closure. A public meeting of a Trust hospital is often a forum for lively discussion. As can be imagined, if the business of the day is concerned with, for example, the closure of a ward, the interested parties, including the general public, are likely to become involved in some bitter and fiery exchanges.

Trust hospitals are not completely 'free' to act as they wish. First, they are well advised to work closely with their major purchasers to ensure that the needs of the local community are satisfied, particularly as the trusts are dependent on the funds received from these contracts. Trusts accept a responsibility to provide the services specified in the contracts and identified by the purchasers. Failure to do this may result in loss of contracts in future negotiations to other competing providers.

Second, the trusts are accountable to the NHS Management Executive which ensures that the trusts are expected to recognise government priorities, and consequently the NHS management executive exerts a very real influence on the services the trusts provide. Third, trusts must be aware of the policies of the NHS policy board and be willing to incorporate these policies into their strategic planning. It can therefore be argued that the government exerts a considerable control over the activities of NHS trusts. The incorporation of trusts into the NHS has not been without criticism. Some critics have suggested that purchasers will opt for cheaper services rather than better services. Published 'league tables' of trust performances tend to concentrate on number and speed of patients treated, rather than quality of treatment, probably because these figures are easier to quantify. Many health workers still feel uncomfortable at the philosophy of 'making money' out of ill health. Also, in a market of competition, some trusts are likely to be successful whereas others are likely to fail. Failed trusts face restricted services and closures (O'Hara 1996), and their patients are likely to be forced to travel considerable distances in order to access their health care. This situation has potentially disastrous consequences in the case of emergencies.

Successful trusts need to develop a close working relationship with their local commissioning agency and purchasers, since they need to play an active part in meeting the health-care needs of their local community. If a patient is sent to another trust for whatever reason, for example, the local trust does not have the specialities required to treat; the money accompanies the patient, that is the commissioning agency pays the new provider by means of an additional contract. Local trusts accept that certain specialities are outside their field of provision and are not able to claw this money back. They are most unwilling, however, to allow funds to be sent to another provider for a service they are able to provide locally, and so it is in their own best interests to ensure that competing providers do not offer a better, cheaper or quicker service.

A series of recommendations has been introduced within the 'Patient's Charter' which empower the clients of the NHS, making them aware of their rights as well as increasing professional accountability. It is expected that these recommendations will improve the quality of the service. Examples of the recommendations are:

- Ninety per cent of patients should not expect to wait for longer than 30 minutes before being seen
- In accident and emergency departments, 90% of patients should receive medical assessment within 5 minutes of entering the department
- Cancelled operations should be rescheduled within 1 month. Where this is not possible the Health Commissioning agency may be forced to use private providers as an alternative.

These recommendations have placed a greater accountability than ever before on professionals and managers in the NHS, though implementation has not always been without difficulty and benefits to clients have not always been clear (Allsop 1995:191).

GP Contracts

Another major change in the delivery of services as a direct result of the NHS act was in the provision of primary health services. General practitioners who cared for more than 9000 patients were invited to apply to become fundholders. (The figure was more recently reduced to 7000 patients.) As fundholders, the GPs received a budget from the RHA, and were therefore able to exert greater control and autonomy over the services they provided and purchased from secondary health-care providers.

Currently, **fundholding General Practitioners** (FHGPs) are effectively providers of primary care and purchasers of secondary care. They run their practices, employ staff and pay their wages. Most practices employ a practice manager to manage the business and financial aspects of their work. These managers are often business people with a financial background, rather than health professionals. FHGPs can purchase secondary services from a range of providers including the **independent sector** as well as NHS trusts. Patients can be referred to a trust in another part of the country if they so wish, and if the patient is likely to benefit, for example by receiving a shorter waiting time for an operation. Because of this flexibility of **contract**, local NHS trusts are willing to work with the

**Case
study 10.2**

Hazel is 24 years old. She is very excited as she suspects she may be pregnant with what she hopes will be her first baby and, consequently, she makes an appointment to see her GP. Her elder sister, Jill, advises Hazel to take a urine specimen to the health centre and informs her that the GP will send the specimen to the local NHS trust hospital. She cautions Hazel that she will have to wait a few days for the results. When Hazel visits the GP she is surprised that the practice nurse produces a slide pregnancy-test kit and is delighted when she shows Hazel the positive results within 3 minutes. Jill is equally amazed by this quick result.

This is an example of the changes that have occurred in routine diagnosis since 1990. Many GP practices are now willing to perform a number of basic diagnostic tests, such as urine testing, cholesterol testing, glucose testing and pregnancy testing. There are a number of benefits, e.g. the client receives a quicker service and the GP is able to control the costs of diagnostic and pathology services. However, there are problems, e.g. a range of services which pathology departments traditionally provide are no longer required. This could result in staff reductions and redundancies within these departments.

commissioning agencies to ensure that the secondary care needs of the local FHGPs are met. This suggests that FHGPs are able to provide a better service for their patients than non-fundholders (Baggott 1994).

FHGPs can buy a range of services from their providers. These include:

- diagnostic services, e.g. pathology, blood tests
- drugs
- day care facilities.

In addition, FHGPs perform some of their own diagnostic testing, for example urine testing and pregnancy testing. This allows them to provide a quicker and cheaper service than non-fundholders, who must use the facilities of the local trust. Some FHGPs also perform minor operations, again reducing the waiting time for their clients.

FHGPs are able to draw up contracts with a provider for a service they predict their patients will need. These predictions are based on local knowledge, research and previous requirements. The contract is a formal agreement in which the FHGP and the provider establish the number of operations to be carried out. These contracts may be:

1. Block contracts. These contracts are paid on an annual basis. The GP assesses how many operations she or he will need during the next year and pays in advance for access to these services which the provider agrees to provide.

2. Cost per case contracts. These contracts usually involve a relatively rare procedure and are often quite expensive. The FHGP contracts with a provider on a single-case basis.
3. Additional contractual referrals. DHAs are able to purchase these contracts on behalf of a FHGP for a service which is not covered by the GP contracts. (These contracts are also used for specialist services which local providers do not cover, e.g. spinal injuries and serious burns cases.)

There are certain services which an FHGP cannot purchase from a provider. These services remain outside the contracting abilities of the FHGP and include:

- maternity services
- accident and emergency services
- psychiatry services and other services for the mentally ill
- services for the elderly.

A major criticism of the development of fundholding for GPs has been the observation that a two-tier system of primary health care has been introduced, in which patients who are cared for by an FHGP receive a better service than those cared for by non-fundholders, since the former have greater options and faster through-put (Baggott 1994). The Labour Party is particularly antagonistic to this and before the 1997 General Election vowed to replace fundholding if it was successful in the election. A further criticism suggested that FHGPs would not welcome high-risk expensive clients such as elderly patients, though Glennerster et al (1992) dispute this, stating that there is no evidence to support this view. The hard evidence of the 1990s is that more and more people are being treated by a fundholding GP, including patients of GPs with small practices and small numbers of patients, who are entitled to join together to form a consortium, and hence apply for and acquire fundholding status.

Reflection point 10.3	Consider the extent to which clients are likely to receive a better service if their GP is a fundholder.
	In what particular areas of the service do you think the clients of non-fundholders are likely to be disadvantaged?

Fundholding appears to offer practices a greater autonomy in how they manage their services, and patients of fundholders do have a greater choice in terms of the service they receive. However, it should be noted that the FHGPs are not completely free to run the service as they wish. The health service commissions, formed by the union of the DHA and the FHSA, play an important role in the provision of primary health services, assessing the needs of the local community and setting priorities as well as dealing with complaints. The commission is therefore able to exert a very real influence on the provision of primary services of GPs whether fundholding or non-fundholding, and it is expected that they will now have a greater overview of health service provision than ever before. This should ensure that links between primary and secondary health are more closely forged. The Health Service commission will encourage GPs to take note of government policies and initiatives and provide their services accordingly. This in part explains the willingness of GP practices to improve their preventative strategies, e.g. the provision of Well-Men and Well-Women clinics etc. in accordance with government initiatives such as the White Paper 'The Health of the Nation' (DoH 1992).

GPs did not escape the need for professional accountability and, in addition to the Patient's Charter, many practices established their own charter setting out their intentions and good working practices and expressing client rights. Most charters also set out clients' obligations and the charters were seen as a two-way agreement between doctor and client. The accountability of GPs placed primary care close to a crisis situation in 1995 when it became obvious that many GPs were finding it impossible to meet the requirements of the Patient's Charter. Within localities, GPs from different practices began to work together to provide the out-of-hours services needed to meet the requirements, whilst allowing GPs the opportunity to avoid an impossible workload.

Activity 10.5

Review a copy of a GP practice charter. List any special services the practice offers, e.g. Well-Men and Well-Women clinics, minor surgery, etc. How has the practice developed since 1990? Speculate on the extent to which the fundholding or non-fundholding status of the surgery is a significant influence on the range and type of services offered.

Significant Changes in Health-Care Provision

The major impact of the NHS Act has been to introduce competition into the delivery of health services and to establish a 'mixed economy of care'. This mixed economy is made up of providers from the **statutory sector** and the independent sector, delivering their services to NHS purchasers. (See the section on 'The NHS and Community Care Act' on p 205.)

Statutory provision is established by law. It is paid for by taxation and National Insurance provision and includes the health authorities and NHS trusts. The services provided include hospital services and social security benefits. Private provision is the province of profit-making organisations. It offers a viable alternative to statutory health care for many people living in the UK but, as it is an expensive alternative, many people are unwilling to pay for this option. The **voluntary sector** and informal sector are extremely important and influential sectors of health and care provision in the community but have a more limited role in the hospital sector, although some charitable organisations, e.g. Women's Royal Voluntary Service (WRVS), do exert a substantial influence in hospital catering. Advice agencies and phone lines on specific diseases play a considerable role in the understanding of health care and coping with illness. Nevertheless, for all these options the delivery of treatment in the UK is generally provided by organisations or individuals from the statutory or private sectors. Purchasers or commissioning agencies purchase health care from both sectors. These services are purchased on behalf of the local population using research statistics and previous knowledge to predict the health requirements of local people. These assessments are a very important part of the purchasing role. The purchasers then negotiate contracts with the providers. NHS purchasers, e.g. commissioning agencies and FHGPs, can purchase services from the independent sector if they wish. As Baggott observes: 'Private health care may be purchased out of public funds' (Baggott 1994:114). However, local commissioning agencies do tend to use their local trusts wherever possible and the use of other providers is an unlikely scenario. This is possibly best explained by traditional links. If purchasers are happy with the services provided by their local trust, there is less likelihood of looking for cheaper, quicker alternatives elsewhere. Moreover, patients traditionally expect to receive their operations locally whenever possible, and GPs seem less willing to dispatch their patients to distant parts of the UK in order to bring forward the time of their operations.

Throughout the 1990s some DHAs have performed the role of purchaser whereas others have been providers of health care. If the local district hospital has been successful in its application for trust status, the hospital takes on the role of provider and the DHA becomes the purchaser. However, during this transition, some district hospitals remain which do not possess the self-governing status that trusts do. These are called Direct Managed Units (DMU). Although they are the focus of hospital service delivery and provision, they are not involved in contracting out their services and the DHA remains the provider. Consequently, over the last six years both models of hospital service delivery have been implemented.

In order to increase their purchasing power and to rationalise their services, some DHAs have joined together to make larger commissioning units. These large authorities linked up with the FHSA in 1996 as identified in the section on Trust hospitals. This further increases the overall view of the health-care needs of the population in both the primary and secondary care areas. These authorities are responsible for joint initiatives and they are intended to avoid overlaps. The Health Service Commissions should ensure that links between primary health care and secondary health care are forged and that the overall health-care needs of local populations are identified. The 'Health of the Nation' initiative attempted to raise the profile of preventative health care in the UK, a philosophy which requires the support of both primary and secondary care if it is to succeed in whatever form the Labour government prescribes. At the time of writing it is not clear what approach the Labour government will take.

Activity 10.6	Contact your local CHC and request a copy of the most recent annual report and public health report of the commissioning/purchasing authority for your district.
	Try to discover the recent strategies in your district aimed at meeting the 'Health of the Nation' targets.
	Identify the social and environmental factors that influence the achievement of the 'Health of the Nation' targets.
	Gauge the significance of these factors in meeting 'Health of the Nation' targets.

The Health of the Nation

The government White Paper of 1992 'The Health of the Nation' (DoH 1992) was an important document for health service workers, as it caused a shift in emphasis on the way they worked throughout the first half of the 1990s. The government proposal set out targets which health providers and purchasers were expected to work together to achieve. Most of the targets were within the area of preventative diseases. In other words, considerable progress could be made in achieving the targets if the authorities made a shift in emphasis of their health-care strategies to preventative health, developing their health promotion, health education and awareness strategies as well as improving their diagnostic, medical and surgical skills. The document set out targets which specifically aim to reduce the mortality rates in certain areas. For example:

- coronary heart disease
- strokes
- breast cancer
- suicide
- accidents.

Moreover, the targets were very specific. For example, in terms of heart disease the White Paper suggested authorities should reduce mortality rates of clients aged under 65 years by 40% by the year 2000; for clients aged 65–74 years the reduction was set at 30% by 2000. The paper identified risk factors that should be addressed, e.g. diet and nutrition, smoking, obesity and alcohol consumption. Targets were also set for this area. In the case of smoking, the rate of smoking in both sexes by the year 2000 was to be reduced to less than 20%. The strategies used to meet these targets were not specified within the paper since local autonomy was seen as important in addressing these problems. Health Commissions, purchasers and local providers were expected to work together to meet the targets using local knowledge, skills and expertise. The strategies employed by different DHAs have been very varied and innovative. One DHA decided to purchase more angiograms for coronary artery bypass grafts to reduce the number of deaths by heart disease, as well as developing a more effective health promotion and screening package for cancer, covering lung, breast, skin and cervical cancers. Another DHA developed a very vivid health promotion package promoting breast feeding, rubella immunisation and the dangers of smoking for maternity cases. A third DHA concentrated on mentally ill clients, providing support accommodation within the community and a 24-hour crisis response, together with a study on postnatal depression. Obviously the range of interventions was very varied as the White Paper offered considerable scope for creativity, although there has been some criticism of the level of financial backing to the initiative. Although innovation and creativity are fundamentally important features in order for health services and their staff to tackle the challenges set by the 'Health of the Nation' target, a general improvement in healthy living and quality of life expectancy requires not only health services to be proactive but for the general public to be receptive to change. The improvement in health education and health promotion strategies is a starting point, but encouraging the citizens of the UK to access these packages and then to incorporate their suggestions into a healthier lifestyle is not likely to be easy for a number of reasons.

First, the citizens of the UK have come to accept the NHS as a treatment service. Although information in the form of, for example, posters and leaflets as well as individual advice can readily be accessed from one's local health centre, the majority of people visit their GP or hospital to be treated. Encouraging clients to use the service for preventative measures, such as information gathering, is likely to be very difficult and, if successful, to add to the GPs heavy workload and to the practice budget. Second, the citizens of the UK must fundamentally change their view on health. They must recognise the need to become involved in their own health and take responsibility for it. This requests that each citizen takes ownership for her or his fitness and undertakes to live as healthy a lifestyle as possible. In other words, local health service providers can work together to target specific groups to stop smoking, for example, as part of the health of the nation targets to reduce the rates of cancer; however, unless a large enough response is induced within the target group, and the citizens are amenable to change, the strategy will ultimately be unsuccessful. Moreover this change must not be transient. Individuals must continue with their healthy lifestyle and not give it up. Such a strategy is not easy to maintain. As Richard Smith notes: 'The easy part of strategic planning is devising a strategy. The difficult part is making it happen' (Smith et al 1992:6). He identifies sustained motivation as a problem area: 'The problem after implementation is to sustain motivation and commitment' (Smith 1992:7).

Other participants are also needed to contribute to a successful health promotion strategy. The government must be prepared to provide additional resources if these become necessary, and the media can play a vital role in reaching as wide an audience as possible. Obviously the success of the 'Health of the Nation' strategies was not easy to achieve, and health promotion innovations by the Minister of Public Health in the Labour government elected in 1997, in what ever form they take, will also be faced with difficulties and challenges. Nevertheless, a serious commitment by the government and by a variety of other interested parties could bring about real advances in the prevention of ill-health and ultimately prove to be an efficient and cost-effective model of health-care delivery. This is particularly so when the alleviated suffering of those for whom ill-health is avoided, is included as part of the overall cost analysis.

Discussion question 10.1

Many experts on and informed critics of the NHS observe that rationing of health care in a variety of forms is a fundamental characteristic of health service provision in the UK (Ham 1992, Klein 1995).

How far do you agree or disagree with these observations about rationing?

To what extent do you consider that the rationing of services was a 'characteristic' in the NHS in 1948?

Beyond inflation, what are the reasons for the ever-increasing costs of the NHS from 1948 to the present time?

New Innovations of the Labour government

A Labour government, often referred to as 'New Labour', was elected on 1 May 1997. Its General Election Manifesto committed an incoming Labour government to 'the historic principle' that there would be a new

NHS, and access to the service would be based on need, not ability to pay. The manifesto suggested that primary care would take a leading role and that GP fundholding – abhorrent to the Labour Party in opposition, since it was believed to be responsible for creating a two-tier service in which patients of non-fundholding GPs were disadvantaged – would be abolished. The Labour party also pledged to introduce a Minister for Public Health, and to set new overall goals for improving the health of the nation. Included in this public health package was a willingness to ban tobacco advertising (Labour Party Manifesto 1997:20–21).

Early indication that the government was serious in fulfilling its election promises were the details on a ban on cigarette advertising, introduced in the Queen's Speech, and the appointment of Tessa Jowell as the Minister for Public Health, supplementing the position of Minister of Health filled by Frank Dobson. On 7 August 1997 the *Health Service Journal* noted that on day 74 of the new administration the Department of Health hosted an anti-smoking summit, in which a ban on smoking in public places and raising the legal age for the purchase of cigarettes to 18 were two of the issues discussed (HSJ, 7 August 1997:13).

Two days later Frank Dobson told health authorities and trusts to operate single waiting lists for fundholding and non-fundholding GPs, in line with the Labour Party Manifesto commitments to remove the two-tier system of general practice (HSJ, 6 August 1997:13).

These early indicators whetted the appetite of health service writers and critics who eagerly awaited the White Paper entitled 'The New NHS: Modern: Dependable' which was published in December 1997.

The White Paper identified a number of key themes designed to develop the existing strengths of the NHS and to remove the weaknesses. These themes included:

- The introduction of a 24-hour nurse helpline to be piloted in March 1998 using three helplines in specific localities and to encompass the whole country by 2000.
- One billion pounds to be saved by removing the internal market and reducing excessive bureaucracy which would be channelled into patient care.
- An NHS information superhighway to be introduced which would ensure patients would spend less time waiting for, e.g., prescriptions and some hospital test results.
- A fast track cancer service to be introduced, in which everyone with suspected cancer would be able to see a specialist within 2 weeks of their GP requesting an appointment
  (DoH 1997:4–7).

The White Paper identified a number of key changes in health service delivery:

- The NHS would work towards improvement in health as well as treatment of sick people.
- The government would tackle the issue of ill-health and inequality, demanding that the NHS work locally with providers of social care, housing, education and employment.
- The public health needs of the citizens of the UK would be addressed, details of which would be enclosed in the forthcoming Green Paper 'Our Healthier Nation' (DoH, forthcoming).
- The internal market would be scrapped and be replaced by 'integrated care', a 10-year programme in which doctors and nurses would be the focus of a local health service aimed at meeting local health-care needs.

The White Paper emphasised a 10-year evolutionary change rather than radical upheaval and reform, and that access to the NHS would be based on need. The new service would be a development of the old philosophy with new technology. The word 'patient' was reintroduced to the literature replacing the more economically loaded 'client' and 'consumer' (DoH 1997).

Perhaps the most important question which arises from a study of the White Paper is whether or not the proposed changes are achievable and of value. This question is perhaps an obvious one, but in view of the limited success of the many attempts by successive Labour and Conservative governments to improve the NHS over the past 30 years, it is necessarily a poignant issue. The government is right to emphasise the extensive demands on the NHS during the 1990s. Within the White Paper these are identified under the broad headings of 'growing public expenditure, medical advances and demographic changes' (DoH 1997:7). Certainly NHS staff recognise these constraints and do believe that the Labour government is dedicated to the improvement of quality of the service. Most NHS staff support the removal of extensive bureaucracy and the reintroduced notion of the 'patient' rather than the redundant 'client'.

Obviously the support of the majority of staff is a great advantage to the Labour government, but support is not sufficient in itself to bring about change. Funding remains a key issue and the government is sticking with its manifesto promise of not raising taxes, just as its Conservative predecessor did not. The government also rejects a charge-based system, expecting to raise the necessary additional funding from efficiency drives, particularly from reduction in the bureaucracy of the internal market system. An evaluation as to whether or not this is successful will have to be made at a later date. Certainly previous efficiency drives have not been particularly successful within the NHS, but perhaps in the 1990s health-care workers and patients are more aware of the need to use limited resources sparingly and appropriately, and have acquired a greater incentive in accepting cheaper options and avoiding waste than those of the 1970s and 1980s.

The government suggests that demographic pressures can be over-stated and identifies the provision of health care for an additional 100 000 people over-85 as a minimal problem. Surely this is over simplifying demographic issues. The NHS will not only be concerned with meeting the needs of the over-85s but also the increasing number of over-75s and over-65s for that matter, all of which are likely to place a substantial demand on health service resources. Moreover the suggestion that the NHS has coped with greater demographic changes in the past and larger numbers of over-85 patients have been catered for is open to question and debate. Many would say that the NHS has only coped by employing volunteers and developing the informal sector, depending upon friends and family to provide many traditional health and care services. Also, demography is concerned with unemployment figures and changing patterns of disease. Although recent figures have pointed to an improvement in unemployment statistics, the existing level of unemployment is still likely to have an effect on government policy for some time to come, and the cushion that the NHS has experienced in successfully combating infectious diseases has recently felt a little less comfortable, not only with the threat of HIV/AIDS but also with the identification of a diverse range of new infectious diseases including legionnaire's disease and BSE, and the recognition of resistant strains of known pathogens such as tuberculosis and multiple resistant staphylococcus aureus (MRSA). At least in the case of BSE the Labour government has taken a more proactive stance than its predecessor by, for example, banning 'beef on the bone' in December 1997. This stance did not meet with universal approval, however, as many consumers saw the stance as government interference. Whilst the government's plans to make better use of its resources (DoH 1997:8) is a praiseworthy suggestion, and most health commentators would agree that the internal market has driven up administration costs, this chapter has identified a number of initiatives which have been designed and introduced with the said intention of improving efficiency, mostly with limited success. Although the Government intention of re-allocating £1 billion from bureaucracy to patient care will receive wide support, the consequences of this reallocation will need to be seen before an underlying scepticism is laid to rest.

Sensibly, the government has not abandoned the idea of appropriate rationing. Screening for prostate cancer is identified (DoH 1997:8–9) as being financially non-viable. Where sufficient research is carried out and the benefits clearly demonstrated to be of little value, the rejection of health practices will be more acceptable than rejection based purely on financial parameters.

The government's claim that for the first time in the history of the NHS 'clinical and financial responsibility will be aligned' (DoH 1997:9) will not completely convince health service critics who recall the attempts of the 1974 reorganisation to marry contributions of health service treasurers with a range of professional practitioners in the laborious concept of 'consensus management'. In a more streamlined NHS in which all parties should be more aware of financial constraints, the government is probably right to expect that decision making involving clinicians and accountants will be more effective and responsible.

The commitment of the government to build on successes within the NHS and to reject the failures rather than to plump for a complete reform seems an eminently sensible approach which is likely to attract support from health-care workers who, having experienced a considerable round of changes during the past few years, should appreciate a period of consolidation. Nevertheless, what the government views as successes may not totally align itself with all health workers. The White Paper's repeated assurances that GPs will maintain their independent status may not satisfy all GPs who are expected to become a central part of the integrated system within a primary care group. Non-fundholding GPs in particular, who have resisted the financial options of fundholding within the internal market, may view this involvement as giving them less choice than before, since all GPs are now expected to form part of the partnership which will be the primary care group, and there are no opportunities for opting out.

The very notion of partnership, though a recognised ideal of many involved in the delivery of health and social care, has not been easy to achieve in practice. The government is right to suggest that a system requiring the contributions of not only a wide variety of health professionals but also professionals from the local authorities, housing, education and unemployment will take time to gel before effective designing of local health-improvement programmes is experienced throughout the UK. The structure of primary care groups, for example, with 4 identified phases of development, will at least allow local professionals, doctors and nurses the breathing space to adapt to the new system and to contribute to it at the appropriate level, for example at level 1, as a support to the local authority in commissioning care for those with little experience, or at level 4 for those who have the experience and confidence to become free-standing bodies with accountability to the health authorities. This at least suggests that the government is committed to its proposals for evolutionary development of the service and aware that progression is likely to vary from locality to locality.

The White Paper clearly identifies a shift within health policy from the previous focus on financial constraints to one in which quality becomes the major drive. The development of national standards and guidelines and local measures to enable NHS staff to take responsibility for improving quality are stated goals within the White Paper (DoH 1997:18). Whilst this fundamental change in philosophy is likely to gain considerable support among practitioners, there is still likely to be a degree of scepticism and uncertainty that such quality improvements can be attainable without a considerable increase in additional health-care funding. As the government is opposed to increasing taxes, this additional funding is expected to come from efficiency drives. Whilst the saving of £1 billion by removal of bureaucracy and the extension of strategic planning cycles (from 1 year to 3 years) are likely improvements for the new NHS, it remains to be seen if sufficient savings can be made to finance the new system and improve quality as the White Paper intends. Any additional funds gathered in this way will need to be used very carefully if the already damaged morale of health service staff is not to be further harmed by the ominous suggestion of a new organisation to address shortcomings (DoH 1997:18). This identification of public accountability may lead to reprimands for 'shortcomings' and ultimately closures and redundancies. However unpalatable these may appear, at least if the underlying philosophy is quality of care and not financial gain, the bitter pill of rationalisation may be easier to swallow.

The White Paper sets out 6 key principles:

- to renew the NHS as a genuinely national service
- to make the delivery a matter of local responsibility
- to get the NHS to work in partnership and to forge greater links with local authorities
- to drive efficiency based on performance and to cut bureaucracy
- to guarantee excellence in quality of care
- to rebuild public confidence
   (DoH 1997:11).

All these principles are praiseworthy objectives. Whether they are attainable within the 10 years the government has allocated to the NHS developments remains to be seen. Indeed, whether the government itself remains for two periods of office obviously depends upon the result of the next General Election, and that may be influenced by the success or otherwise of the NHS development during the first period in office. The principles are not entirely new. The search for efficiency in the NHS has been a fundamental aim throughout its long history, particularly since 1970; but all too often this has led to greater bureaucracy and not less, whilst decentralisation, the development of primary care and local provision with increased accountability have been promoted by successive Conservative governments since 1980. The need for successful partnerships between health professional and social care practitioners of local authorities were identified as early as the 1974 reorganisation and have gained substantial momentum since 1990 and the development of the internal market. These partnerships have not always been successful because of a basic lack of co-ordination between a diverse group of professionals.

The White Paper successfully identifies areas of great need within the NHS. It reflects upon the contributions of many NHS staff and identifies a necessary change in philosophy from a financially-driven service to a quality-driven service, mindful of financial constraints. It recognises strengths and weaknesses in the current system and broadly identifies a view of the future which incorporates these strengths and scraps the weaknesses. What the White Paper lacks is specific details of how these aims are to be achieved. On the one hand, it is commendable to prescribe a partnership between health professionals and a range of other contributors to health including the local authorities, housing, education and unemployment, and it is also fine to state that local professionals will have the autonomy to provide health services for local people; however, on the other hand, detailed plans of how these innovations are to be achieved are not included. The contradictory goal of health service staff being able to balance quality and excellence within financial constraints and budgets may remain unattainable even after 10 further years of development.

Summary

By studying this chapter and working through the activities and reflections, you will have become aware of the amount of change and restructuring that has occurred within the NHS since its inception as a tripartite system in 1948. These changes can be seen as the attempts of consecutive Conservative and Labour governments to control the increasing cost of the statutory health services. The desire to control this increase in public expenditure has become more urgent as unemployment has risen, and the number of elderly and very elderly people living in the UK has increased. Moreover, the development of modern medical technology has added greatly to the cost of health service delivery and is likely to continue in this manner. The political debate on how to control health service expenditure is likely to continue throughout the coming decade.

You will be aware that the recent initiative to control NHS expenditure – the 'NHS and Community Care Act' of 1990 – has had a major impact on health and care provision in the 1990s.

In 1997 a Labour government was elected in the UK; this government is committed to improvement in public health and the comprehensive provision of health services for everyone regardless of ability to pay. Obviously the potential of this health policy is exciting and the success or lack of success of the Labour administration will be keenly scrutinised during the remainder of the decade.

This chapter has concentrated on the NHS Act, exploring the developments in health provision, particularly in the hospital sector.

Further Reading

Allsop J 1995 Health policy and the NHS: towards 2000, 2nd edn. Longman, London
This is a very useful text which will give you more details on the reorganisations of the NHS.

Klein R 1995 The new politics of the NHS, 3rd edn. Longman, London
This is an essential text for anyone who is interested in the political decision making of health services and in analysing rationing of health care.

Baggott R 1994 Health and health care in Britain. Macmillan, London
This is an excellent all round text in which the purchaser and provider split and the 'mixed economy of care' are covered very well and in a way that most readers will find easy to access and understand.

References

Allsop J 1995 Health policy and the NHS: towards 2000, 2nd edn. Longman, London
Alaszewski A, Tether P, Macdonnell H 1981 Another dose of managerialism? Commentary 15a. Social Sciences and Medicine 1: 5–15
Annual report of the United Health Commission 1995 Grimsby DHA, Scunthorpe DHA and FHSA
Baggott R 1994 Health and health care in Britain. Macmillan, London
BMA 1930 A general medical service for the Nation. British Medical Association, London
Department of Health (DoH) 1989 Working for patients. Cmnd. 555. HMSO, London
Department of Health (DoH) 1992 The health of the nation. HMSO, London
Department of Health (DoH) 1997 The new NHS: Modern: Dependable. Cmnd. 3807. HMSO, London
Department of Health (DoH), forthcoming, Our healthier nation. HMSO, London
Glennerster H, Owens P, Matsaganis M 1992 A footholding for fundholding. King's Fund, London
Griffiths R 1983 The NHS management enquiry report. DHSS, London
Ham C 1992 Health policy in Britain. The politics and organisations of the National Health Service, 3rd edn. Macmillan, London
Ham C, Robinson R, Benzeval M 1990 Health check. King's Fund, London
Klein R 1983 The new politics of the NHS. Longman, London
Klein R 1995 The new politics of the NHS, 3rd edn. Longman, London
Labour Party Manifesto 1997 Because Britain deserves better. The Labour Party, London
Levitt R 1979 The reorganised National Health Service, 2nd edn. Croom Helm, London
Ministry of Health 1920 Interim report on the future provision of medical & allied services. HMSO, London. Cmnd. 693 (The Dawson report)
Newfield M 1941 A real medical service. Picture Post 10(1)

NAHA 1987 Autumn survey. National Association of Health Authorities

Nicholl J, Beeby W, Williams B 1989 Roles of the private sector in elective surgery in England and Wales 1986. British Medical Journal 298: 243–247

O'Hara S 1996 The NHS past, present and future. Gazette of the Institute of Biomedical Sciences. November: 605–607

Public health report of the United Health Commission 1995 Grimsby DHA and Scunthorpe DHA

Report of the Royal Commission on the NHS 1979 Chairman Sir Alec Merrison. Cmnd. 7615. HMSO, London

Smith R et al 1992 The health of the nation: the BMJ view. BMJ publications, London

Thatcher M 1993 The Downing Street Years. HarperCollins, London

11 Caring in a Mixed Economy

John Clayton

Key concepts
- What is community?
- Why community care now?
- An outline of community care
- The Carers (Recognition and Services) Act (1995)
- Informal carers
- The significance for nursing

The provision of health and care services in local communities has tended to be pluralistic, i.e. a great variety of services have been provided by a great variety of different organisations and individuals. For this reason the provision has often been criticised as being fragmented and lacking co-ordination. Recent governments have attempted to address these issues whilst searching for efficient and cost-effective models of delivery. These areas of study form the basis of this chapter.

What is Community? ˙

The term **community** means different things to different people and, in attempting to arrive at a definition, it is reasonable to suggest that the term has a very specific meaning for health and care workers. Most general definitions of 'community' will incorporate the idea of a locality or small area where people share common interests. Further definitions may advance the notion that these interests are social, cultural or even political with an idea of ownership. The ownership of the community indicates some feeling of possession by the members of the community.

These definitions of community can be applied to the field of health care. Health and care are often seen as possessions by the people of the UK, who therefore demonstrate a degree of ownership of the services.

The ownership is shared with other interested parties, that is other clients and service providers. In terms of provision, community and health-care services fall broadly into two inter-related and non-exclusive fields:

- Health care as provided by primary care teams.
- Social care is commissioned and provided by the Local Authority Social Services Department (LASSD).

Community health care covers a wide area of provision. Broadly speaking, the professional with the greatest autonomy is the general practitioner (GP). The services are co-ordinated from clinics, health centres, GP surgeries and GP practices. A number of different professions can be expected to contribute to the provision including nurses, health visitors and midwives; see Chapter 10, sections on 'GP contracts' (p 211) and 'Significant changes in healthcare provision' (p 214). Dentists, opticians and pharmacists working in the community, contribute to the overall provision of community health care.

In the 1990s, government priorities, which aimed at developing the independent sector of health services, have opened up the market for private providers such as chiropractors and chiropodists, as well as voluntary providers and help lines. Although official rhetoric in the 1990s has tended to imply that the Conservative government was profoundly concerned about vulnerable people and their need for community care, many workers believed that this concern was a myth and that the market economy, was essentially designed to offer the government cheap options of community care and tighter control on public spending.

They were sceptical of the apparent good intentions of the Community Care Act (1990) and the preceding White Paper, 'Caring for People' (DoH 1989c):

> 'Community care means providing the services and support which people who are affected by problems of ageing, mental illness, mental handicap or physical or sensory disability need to be able to live as independently as possible in their own homes, or in homely settings in the community.'
> (DoH 1989c:3)

This scepticism was not totally unfounded. The Conservative government had made no secret of its desire to control public spending. As early as 1979, in its first year in office, the Thatcher government began to introduce policies to tighten public spending. As Thatcher recalls:

> 'Our first task was to make whatever reductions we could for the current financial year 1979–80.'
> (Thatcher 1993:49)

The first strategy was to raise prescription charges for the first time in eight years. The early indications were that the Conservative government would hit health and social care services to satisfy its monetarist policies.

Although the ultimate reason for the shift towards community care in 1990 was almost certainly economic, there can be no argument that the choice of provision for 'well-to-do' elderly clients was considerably increased within the community with a rapidly advancing private sector allowing a greater number and variety of private health-care professionals to 'make a living'.

Community social care now includes a variety of services for vulnerable groups of people, namely children and families, elderly people, people with mental health problems or learning disability and people with physical disability. These services are part of the 'mixed economy of care' which means that they may be provided by the private and voluntary sectors as well as the statutory sector. The services are co-ordinated by the LASSD, and are provided by social workers or commissioned by the social services department. The range of provider is very diverse and includes, in addition to the private sector and voluntary sectors, a growing number of informal carers. These services are often referred to as the 'personal social services'.

A major priority of the Conservative government of the 1990s was to encourage the care and treatment of clients within their own home, or in short-stay institutions which were modelled on a home environment. This priority was a central feature of the Community Care Act of 1990, with the prime objective being the replacement of long-stay institutions such as mental hospitals, with home-based community care. Health-care clients receiving hospital treatment were also encouraged to convalesce in their own homes as soon as possible, although this is another area of policy which did not go uncriticised. There was criticism that many clients were sent home to recuperate too quickly and without the necessary home care, and that the onus was on the families to provide this support. As family members could not be expected to possess the nursing expertise and skills required, the level of care the clients received was often insufficient. Moreover, criticism of the lack of co-ordination between the health authorities and local authority social services departments was not uncommon. The Carers (Recognition and Services) Act 1995, seeks to address some of these criticisms (see below).

Despite these difficulties within the field of health and social care, 'the community' has become the major area of development in the 1990s. Professional practitioners employed within the areas of health and social care are becoming increasingly involved in the provision of support and advice in the care and treatment of clients living within their own homes or in community-based accommodation, which is as close to the home environment as possible. Meredith's definition encompasses many of these ideas:

> 'Community care is helping people who need care and support to live with dignity and as much independence as possible in the community.'
>   (Meredith 1993)

Reflection point 11.1   Think of any clients you know or have been involved with during your work or studies. How do you feel about discharging them from hospital to recover at home? What are the benefits to the client? Are there any issues which concern you about this priority?

Why Community Care Now?

As identified previously, a major priority of the Conservative government of the 1990s was to shift the emphasis from hospital treatment and institutionalisation to care within the community.

This is not, however, a completely new concept. The White Paper 'The Development of Community Care' (1960) and 'The Hospital Plan' of 1962 of Enoch Powell (Conservative Minister of Health) proposed the replacement of long-stay mental institutions by smaller psychiatric units attached to district general hospitals. The move towards community health and social care provision further gained momentum in the 1970s when White Papers for a number of client groups maintained this priority, e.g. 'Better Services for the Mentally Handicapped' (DHSS 1971) and 'Better Services for the Mentally Ill' (DHSS 1975). Community care has remained on the political agenda throughout the 1980s and has regained momentum in the 1990s with the implementation of the policies of the Community Care Act. It is, however, important at this point, to recognise the shift in emphasis of community care in the 1990s. In the 1960s the expectation was that community care would be provided in the community by professional health and social care workers. In the 1990s the expectation is that professional intervention will be minimised and that community care will be provided by 'the community', with greater independence sought for the client. This demands that the society of the UK in the 1990s is 'neighbourly' and that people take an active and philanthropic interest in their friends, neighbours as well as in the community itself, particularly with regard to its vulnerable members. With increase in crime, and with particularly vivid examples of aggression against older people a regular feature in the media, one is entitled to question whether this is the case.

Nevertheless, it is possible to identify a number of reasons for this shift towards a community-based health and social care service, though, broadly speaking, the reasons are economic and of benefit to the government or altruistic and of benefit to the client group.

Throughout the early years of the NHS the emphasis on the development of community services was probably altruistic, since economic issues had not reached the critical levels that were to follow in future developments and governmental policy was aimed at thoroughly resourcing the community care option and providing qualified personnel to deliver it. 'The Hospital Plan' should be seen as a genuine attempt to provide a better service for all client groups, since there was a recognition that institutionalisation was not the most suitable method of care and treatment for clients in general. The White Papers investigating the 'Better services' for mentally handicapped and mentally ill people recognised that clients made better progress if they were treated and cared for in short-stay institutions integrated into the local community. The question of dependence was recognised to be of real importance by care professionals since long-stay institutionalisation led to a greater degree of dependence and removed the client's ability to live as normal a life as possible. Throughout the 1980s independence came to be accepted as a basic client right and the shift to community care was seen as a more appropriate model for client groups to live as normal a way of life as possible.

The development of the informal care sector can be seen as a further initiative in the support of independence, as family members and friends take on an increasing role of health and care provider. The expanded role of family and friends is not without support, as there is a general acceptance among community health and social care providers that clients recover more successfully if they can be returned to their family and friends and be cared for within their own homes. The support of professionals is seen as essential, however, and inadequate professional back-up is a common area of concern and dissatisfaction. Excessive support is also criticised, however, being seen as interference by the family members providing care. Where clients need to stay in hospital, it is accepted that the stay should be as brief as possible and that clients should be allowed to regain their independence quickly.

Another motive for the development of the community health and care services was the expectation that this would be accompanied by a shift of resources away from the hospital services to vulnerable groups, e.g. the elderly and disabled. This redistribution of resources had been a goal of successive governments since the 1970s, and the Community Care Act provided a model by which this could become a reality since funds would need to be directed towards vulnerable clients. Economic restraints, however, have generally demanded that insufficient funds are available to make this a reality. The development of community care does offer clients benefits, but the recent pressure to expand community services has been essentially economic. Demographic changes have been of fundamental importance in the regained momentum to develop community care, since the steady rise in unemployment since 1970 has forced successive governments to look carefully at the way public services are funded. As less money is taken by the exchequer through taxation, and more money is distributed to unemployed people through social security benefits, there is a reduced budget available to other public services and cheaper alternatives of health-care and social-care delivery needed to be identified. Developments in health-care delivery and medical technology have led to a greater number of elderly people (aged over 65 years) and very elderly people (aged over 75 years) in the community. Elderly people tend to be greater users of health care than young people and are more likely to suffer from chronic conditions which cannot be cured but which need prolonged treatment and care, e.g. arthritis, angina, etc. Alternative methods of caring for these clients needed to be cost effective. The introduction of community health and care offers a cheaper alternative to hospitalisation and long-stay care.

The 1980s witnessed an expansion of the voluntary sector and the private sector in the field of health and care. This expansion received government support (see Chapter 10). Clients now have a greater choice than before in health and care provision, particularly those clients who can afford to pay for private health care. For these people the massive increase in private residential homes during the 1980s and 1990s and the opportunity to access a range of private health-care practitioners can contribute to a positive experience of community care. However, as many vulnerable people fall into the lower income categories of British society, their choice is considerably reduced and many private health practitioners and residential homes are outside their price range. Poorer clients have a very much reduced choice of care and their experience of community care is some way short of their expectations and of the aspirations of the Labour government of 1948, with its pledge to provide a comprehensive service, free for all the citizens of the UK, regardless of their ability to pay.

Poorer clients are dependent on the statutory and voluntary sectors for the most part. Within the field of social care particularly, expansion of the voluntary sector has contributed to a more cost-effective community care provision. The expansion of the **informal sector** can be seen as the most cost-effective development of all, since friends and families usually receive no payment for the caring services they provide (although they are able to claim benefits and allowances; see Chapter 10). Largely, on account of these economic issues, the Community Care Act has been heavily criticised. There have been criticisms within the House of Commons that clients are returned to the community too quickly and that potentially dangerous clients who suffer from serious mental illness could be returned to the community with disastrous consequences.

Informal carers must bear the brunt of caring for sick relatives and there has been evidence to suggest that some informal carers are not suitable, for example they may be too young. As Ackers and Fordham identify:

> 'A particular area of concern is the growing number of young carers of school age or below. In 1993, the Carers National Association (CNA) estimated that well over 10 000 children act as primary carers nationwide.'
>   (Ackers & Fordham 1995:126)

The level of professional support offered to informal carers has also been criticised as inadequate, despite this being a key objective of the White Paper 'Caring for People' (DoH 1989c): 'to ensure that service providers make practical support for carers a high priority' and 'assessment of care should take account of the needs of family, friends and neighbours'.

The criticisms illustrated that family members, friends and neighbours were not always receiving the support the White Paper envisaged. In addition, it was recognised that young children, adopting the role of carer, were themselves in need. These serious issues led to the introduction of the Carers (Recognition and Services) Act 1995, which seeks to ensure that specific groups of people (including those aged under 18 years) receive necessary support for the care they provide. (The act is discussed in more detail on p 240.)

Activity 11.1	Visit your nearest library which has a CD-ROM facility. Access the newspapers on the CD-ROM for the years 1993 to the present. Try to find any examples of mentally-ill clients who have been returned to the community with insufficient professional support. What was the outcome?

As you have seen, the care and treatment of clients in the community offers vulnerable people certain benefits. It improves their independence and their prospects of recovery. It should ensure that client groups receive a greater proportion of the funds available to health and social care, and it is likely to offer wealthy clients a greater choice of providers. The benefits to the government are economic. The services are generally a cost-effective alternative, being cheaper than hospital and long-stay care. In the case of informal carers the economic benefits are likely to be greatest. Provided the voluntary and informal carers delivering the services receive sufficient professional support, however, the range of benefits to the client and the economic benefits to the government need not conflict. Indeed, the development of community health and care is likely to offer opportunities for all the sectors of the health and care services to work together. Primary health-care providers work with local hospital trusts more closely than before. The newly formed Health Service Commissioning agencies which combine the powers of the former district health authority (DHA) and the Family Health Services Authority (FHSA) (see Chapter 10 section on NHS Trusts; p 209) should help to ensure this, and professional people will find their job role changing to include work in the hospital and in the community. Professionals whose backgrounds are in the fields of health and the personal social services should also work more closely together, particularly as vulnerable groups of clients often have need of both of these areas of care delivery. The interactions between the health and social care professionals has been and continues to be criticised. *The Observer* newspaper (MacErlean 1997) contained an article which criticised the early discharge of elderly people from hospital wards to social service provision. The article highlighted the problem as: 'Cash starved social services departments approach the end of their financial year just as the demands of elderly clients peak'. The article also identified the problematic funding issues of interactions between the two services:

> 'There is a crucial financial difference between being treated by the NHS and being cared for by the social services. NHS treatment, including aftercare, is free. Social services is means-tested.'
> (MacErlean 1997:22)

This explains the discrepancy which arises when patients/clients are discharged from hospital into social care, for example into residential homes. The client and their family can be faced with a considerable expense while the aftercare is provided by the social services (MacErlean 1997). These fees are often unexpected and, as hospitals attempt to improve throughput of their clients, hospital stays are more likely to be shortened in the future, and more people are likely to be asked to pay for their aftercare.

However, the likelihood is that for the foreseeable future health and social care professionals will continue to work closely together to provide an integrated community care service. Though the Labour Party General Election Manifesto contains little on community care there is a stated commitment that: Labour 'will retain the lead role for primary care' (Labour Party 1997:21) and the Health Secretary Frank Dobson, who was appointed following Labour's 1997 General Election win, told health authorities, local authorities and other parts of the welfare infrastructure that they must work more closely together to manage the pressure of community care with care and compassion (MacErlean 1997:22).

Indeed, some traditional health professions are likely to be employed by the social services, for example occupational therapists, following initial assessment by social workers. The ideal approach to community health and care is multidisciplinary, which is a model allowing all areas of the service to work together. However, the model is not always straightforward to implement as professionals from disparate backgrounds are not always sure of their exact responsibilities or roles within the team. This suggests that additional resources may need to be made available for training and retraining of staff, so that everyone is familiar with the multi-disciplinary approach. The development of skill mixes have been a feature of multidisciplinary work throughout the 1990s and have led to a greater understanding on one's role within team work. Additional resources to ensure that the service provides the greatest benefits to clients might cause the community provision to be a less cost-effective alternative for the government than was originally thought.

An Outline of Community Care

The large number of people providing health and social care services within the community includes:

- professional people employed by the NHS
- professional people employed by local authorities to deliver social care
- private providers
- voluntary providers
- informal carers such as family members and friends.

While recognising this great diversity, this section attempts to give a broad outline of the provision of community care in the UK. However, no attempt is made to cover all the possible providers, or to identify all the possible services available, since the task would be extremely onerous and the services are likely to vary from one local community to another. This section attempts to give you a broad understanding of community care and to make you aware of the pluralistic nature of community provision.

The provision of community care falls into two broad and interrelated areas:

- Community health care, sometimes referred to as 'primary' health care, and
- Community social care, sometimes referred to as the 'personal social services'.

Community health care involves the treatment and prevention of physical and mental illness within local communities. The services were formerly co-ordinated by the Family Health Services Authority (FHSA) (see section 'What is community?'; p 227). Since April 1996 the FHSA and DHA have combined to form the Health Service Commissioning Agency, with an expanded role in the purchasing of primary and secondary health care within a specific locality. These purchasing authorities obviously have a considerable power in establishing which health services are established and expanded within local communities.

GPs are the major providers of primary health care. They employ staff to work in the practice, e.g. receptionists and practice nurses, and the services are delivered from their practice, surgery or health centre. The services are extremely varied but can include minor surgery, the prescribing of drugs, counselling, and preventative measures such as immunisations and screening. The role of GPs has changed since the White Paper of 1986 entitled 'Promoting Better Health' (DoH 1989a) which essentially increased the role of GPs in the prevention of ill health and the promotion of better health (Ham, 1992). This initiative was accompanied by new contracts for GPs and dentists which included provision for areas of health promotion identified as being significant. These areas included annual check-ups for patients aged 75 or over, plus other work such as immunisation targets, cervical cancer screening and minor operations. The new contracts for dentists also focused on preventative issues, particularly in the provision for children, as dentists received a capitation fee for their child clients instead of payment for the dental services they performed (Ham 1992:52–53).

Another important change in the provision of GP and dental services within the local community was the attempt to increase accountability of the providers by the introduction of the 'Patient's Charter'. Added to this, GP practices and dental surgeries introduced their own charters highlighting their commitment to good working practices, but also identifying the expected client role within the service provision. Although these initiatives were generally viewed as a great improvement with client empowerment being a fundamental right, the workload on GPs in some areas has become excessive and extremely long waiting lists have been cited in some depressed areas within inner cities.

The provision of statutory health care within the community is now the role of primary health care providers with support from the local hospital. The GP practice co-ordinates primary services, including domiciliary visits by the general practice professional care staff. The health authorities employ community nurses to visit clients within the locality to provide a very extensive range of services, which include the essential advice and contact that an ever-increasing number of people need. The role of community nurses is, therefore, fundamental to the success of community care:

> 'Primary care staff, including GPs and community nurses through their contact with users and carers, are in a good position to notice signs of stress, difficulty or rapidly deteriorating health particularly in carers.'
>   (DoH 1996a:9)

Specialist nurses employed by local Trust hospitals are increasingly being employed within the community to visit clients giving advice and support within the areas of their specialty, for example epilepsy, diabetes and Parkinson's disease. Consideration is being given to further developments of the responsibilities of nurses in prescribing, supply and administration of certain medicines which will be informed by the outcome of a Crown Review. This will be enshrined within a legal framework.

The statutory provision of primary health care includes school liaison and health promotion with children, for example receiving regular eye tests, hearing tests and immunisations. Within districts the Health Service Commissioning Authorities, have a substantial purchasing role (see Chapter 10 section on NHS Trusts; p 209), as well as extensive responsibility for overseeing all aspects of health-care need (both primary and secondary). These authorities should help to ensure that local needs are more closely met and that the appropriate services for each specific locality are addressed, with funds being used to purchase the services from the most suitable and cost-effective provider.

Within the field of health care the expansion of the private sector is a very significant development. A range of private providers is available in most districts to offer alternative therapy and treatment to the statutory provision. These providers, which include chiropractors, chiropodists, acupuncturists, osteopaths and homeopaths, charge for their services and, as has been previously highlighted (see Chapter 10), their significance is greater for well-to-do clients who are able to pay for the services directly or by contributing to an insurance-based health plan as a future investment, the company then paying any health-care expenses when needed. Although there has been some interaction between the providers of the statutory sector and the providers of the private sector, the interaction remains limited in most localities, and clients still seem to view the private sector as consisting of 'alternative providers'.

Reflection point 11.2	Consider ways in which the private and public sectors may be expected to show similarities.
	In what areas would you anticipate the most difference?
	Speculate on the ways in which these differences may impact on the experience of care for the patient.

The voluntary sector is less developed in the delivery of health care than in social care, probably because of the level of expertise required in most areas of health-care provision and the legal requirements for qualified status in order to practice. However, the 1980s and 1990s have seen a rapid expansion in help lines and small offices where volunteers with great experience of a particular illness or disease are willing to share their knowledge and skills without charge. Informal carers, including friends and family members who have cared for people with a disease for a number of years, become extremely knowledgeable in coping with some of the disease symptoms and are a valuable source of advice to sufferers and their families.

Case study 11.1

Mr Giles has cared for his wife for 16 years during which she has suffered with Parkinson's disease. During that time Mrs Giles has spent three short sessions in hospital whilst she has been given new drugs to try, so that the staff could monitor her progress. For the remaining time, Mr Giles has cared for his wife alone and the hospital has encouraged Mr and Mrs Giles to experiment with the timing of the drugs and minor adjustments of dosage, to get the best balance for Mrs Giles' needs. Mr and Mrs Giles joined the local Parkinson's group and Mr Giles was surprised when he was asked to talk at a meeting. He did so, and became identified as a useful authority on coping strategies. Although he is too busy caring for his wife to open up a help line, he is pleased to offer his advice and support if approached.

Points to consider:

What are your views on informal advice and help lines?

What other illnesses do you think might benefit from this kind of help?

The most pluralistic of all the areas of health and social care provision is the area of community social care. This is due to the expansion of the private and voluntary sector within this area during the 1980s and 1990s, as well as the expansion of the informal care sector of provision. The range of providers is now extremely diverse and the role of statutory provision within this area is that of a commissioning authority rather than as a major provider. This has meant that the essential role of the major statutory provider, i.e. the LASSD, has changed and, therefore, the role of the social worker has also changed. The LASSD now co-ordinates the social care services within the local community. For this reason they are known as 'enablers' and not providers. Social workers are still involved in provision of certain services as before, for example adoption, fostering, sectioning, assessment of appliances for homes. These are traditional social work roles which still need a qualified social worker. However, some of the traditional roles are no longer viewed as needing professional social work input and LASSD are willing to commission the voluntary and private sector to provide these services if they can demonstrate cost-effectiveness.

The possible range of service providers within a local community is vast, with local support groups and neighbourhood teams supporting the nationwide range of voluntary organisations and charitable organisations such as Age Concern, Mind and Mencap. Indeed, the range of voluntary providers is so extensive that attempts to identify the providers within this sector and their influences would be an enormous task.

'To review the key influences on the work of the voluntary agencies would be an immense task, if the potential influences are legion, the term voluntary agencies also masks an enormous variation.'
(Billis & Harris 1996)

Activity 11.2

What voluntary organisations are available within your community? Pick up a telephone directory, such as Yellow Pages, and make a concise directory of your own. Are there any of the agencies with which you are totally unfamiliar? If so, pay them a visit and find out more about them. You might want to ask them what services they provide, what client groups they care for, how many volunteers work for them, if any of their staff are paid employees and how they acquire their funding.

Voluntary organisations receive their funding from a variety of sources. Larger organisations such as Age Concern are likely to receive a considerable amount of their funding from central government grants and from the local authority. Age Concern is a registered charity, which gives the organisation tax exemptions. The voluntary organisations are able to operate fund-raising events such as sponsored walks and flag days, and receive donations from businesses and individuals.

Private organisations are also heavily involved in the provision of social care. The massive expansion of private residential homes and private nursing homes has been a feature of the service developments since the first half of the 1980s. The LASSD is now able to use the private sector in the same way as the voluntary sector and clients can be housed in private nursing homes by the LASSD who provide the funding for the client. This open market of private, voluntary and statutory provision is part of the 'mixed economy of care', an initiative of the NHS and Community Care Act 1990 (see Chapter 10; p 205). Recent developments within the role of social care provision can be traced back to the Griffiths report of 1988 entitled 'Community Care: Agenda for Action' and the White Paper of 1989 entitled 'Caring for People' (DoH 1989c), which was to become the Community Care Act of 1990. As Baggott identifies, the Griffiths report had three main principles:

- Services should be provided early enough
- Clients should have a greater choice of providers
- People should be cared for within their homes if possible.
(Baggott 1994:229)

These proposals were generally accepted and incorporated into the Community Care Act; and the third proposal had a very clear effect on the largest group of care providers within the UK, i.e. the informal carers. Since more and more people were encouraged to receive their care services within their own home, the need for close family members, friends and neighbours to help more in the provision of care was inevitable. The growth of the informal care sector is perhaps the most rapidly expanding area of all and is explored in the following section.

The role of community care deals specifically with addressing the needs of vulnerable clients, that is elderly people, people with mental health problems or learning disability, people with physical disability and their families. The variety of providers has often raised criticisms of a fragmented and diverse service. The Community Care Act seeks to address these issues by providing greater integration and co-operation between service providers, for example if a social work assessment on a client living at home identifies the need for an occupational therapist to assist the client to cope, the occupational therapist will be employed by the social services to meet the need. The Community Care Act recommends a closer link than before between the provision of health services and the provision of social care. Indeed, clients who are discharged from hospital to their homes may have need of a variety of health and care services. This can create great difficulty with overlap of service provision or, worse, no aftercare whatsoever. Moreover, as health care is free whereas social care is means tested, clients have been made to pay for hospital aftercare delivered in residential homes. It is hoped that as professionals of health and social care begin to work together, the skill mixes will be developed and some of the problems of delivery tackled. However, the funding issues continue to be problematic.

The model of care involving a variety of health and social care professionals is multidisciplinary with a variety of inputs required to meet the diversity of need. In most cases where clients are being cared for at home, sufficient professional support is necessary. These issues have raised some concerns, with the ideal of multidisciplinary approach often a failure in reality, since individuals within large teams are not always sure of their specific role, and the level of support for informal care not always seen as sufficient.

The Carers (Recognition and Services) Act 1995

This Act is of fundamental importance for carers, friends, neighbours and family members who have a substantial commitment for caring for a disabled person within the community. It is concerned with carers who already provide care for friends or family or who are intending to provide such care in the future.

The Act is concerned with specific groups of carers and does not include voluntary or private organisations. The groups targeted are:

- People aged 18 and over who provide or intend to provide a substantial amount of care on a regular basis
- Children and young people (under 18) who provide or intend to provide a substantial amount of care on a regular basis
- Parents who provide or intend to provide a substantial amount of care on a regular basis for a disabled child.
   (DoH 1996a:3)

The carer may or may not live within the same home as the client, but the substantial and regular amount strongly indicates a daily commitment to the client.

Putting the Carers (Recognition and Services) Act into practice necessitates the following procedures. The client is scheduled to have an assessment by the local authority. This assessment is performed by an experienced care manager who will design a care-plan for the client, to meet the needs of the client and to help her or him live as independently as possible within her or his home. (This assessment may be necessary since the client may have recently become disabled, or alternatively the assessment may be a re-assessment since the health of the client may have deteriorated or the circumstances of the care changed.) At the time of this assessment of the client, the carer may also request an assessment by the same care manager as part of the Act. The carer's needs will then be taken into consideration and a care-plan involving the social services, the carer and client will be produced. This care-plan will address the needs of the carer and client and will identify any multidisciplinary support the carer needs. This support might be provided by health professionals, social services, housing or the education department. The role of the care manager is vitally important and experienced staff, with an overall knowledge of all these areas, is needed. The Act is intended to be accessible to all informal carers irrespective of sex, age, race or disability and care managers will be expected to provide written confirmation (or a suitable alternative) of the care-plan to all carers and clients. In this way the Act is designed to meet the needs of both carers and clients and to provide the carers with the necessary professional support. An objective highlighted in the White Paper 'Caring for People' (DoH 1989c). Obviously as the range of illness and disabilities is very wide, each carer and client combination will have very different needs, for example an older person caring for a physically disabled older relative will have different needs from a young carer looking after a relative who has HIV/Aids. Moreover, the circumstances of both are

Case study 11.2	In Chapter 7 the situation of James was highlighted. Here we return to the case of James and move his situation forwards.

51-year-old James was diagnosed as having schizophrenia when he was in his early twenties. Initially, he experienced several lengthy periods of in-patient care within a traditional mental hospital where electroconvulsive therapy and major tranquillisers were the treatment of choice. During this early part of his illness the label 'schizophrenic' became firmly attached and this has stayed with him to the present day. When he was not in hospital James lived with his parents. Because of negative, often hurtful reactions to him by neighbours James became a recluse, only going out during the periods of darkness for short walks.

The time inevitably came when the combination of the 'courtesy stigma', neighbour's complaints and the demands of caring for James became too much for his ageing parents. They began to discuss between themselves and with the community psychiatric nurse the best way of dealing with this increasingly serious situation. A case conference was convened.

Reflect on the various options that could be offered by the social and health services to support James and his parents. Place yourself in the role of James, his mother, his father, and his community psychiatric nurse. It is possible for this short case study to form a basis for a group activity role-playing the case conference.

likely to change over a period of time and so the care-plan will need to be developed.

Although the Act identifies the needs of the carer for professional support and provides a mechanism whereby the carer can seek professional assistance through the request of an assessment, it places an enormous responsibility on care managers and demands that they are completely 'au fait' with all the workings of the **multi-agency** organisations. Moreover, the Act requires that all the partner organisations work together efficiently and that the NHS, local authorities, housing authorities and education authorities are completely aware of their contributions in an extremely diverse set of circumstances. How effective this vitally important piece of legislation is will ultimately depend on the knowledge and co-ordinating skills of care managers and the carefully developed skill mixes of multidisciplinary teams.

The Act, though a new initiative, is seen as a development of current policy:

'The Act links the results of a carer's assessment to the local authority's decision about services to the user. The aim is to encourage an approach

which considers support already available from family, the type of assistance needed by the person being assessed and how and whether the current arrangements for care can sustain the user in the community.'
(DoH 1996a:3)

In the case of the child who provides care, the local authority is expected to consider if the Children Act 1989 applies. It then becomes essential to discover if the young carer 'because of the extent and effect of their caring responsibilities, are children in need' (DoH 1996a:4).

In this way it is expected that young children will not be asked to provide care for disabled parents without appropriate professional support and without their needs being recognised. However, as the assessment of carers as part of the Act is on request at the point of assessment of the client, there still remains a worry that some young carers, ignorant of the Act, will remain unidentified.

Informal Carers

As you will now be aware, the reasons for the development of the informal sector in social care are twofold:

1. The realisation that the sector offers the cheapest option of care available
2. The recognition that institutionalisation is a less successful method of treatment for most people than care in their homes by formal and informal carers.

Informal care is care provided by non-professional carers, usually a friend, a neighbour or most likely of all, a family member of the client. Typically the informal carer is a female family member (Ackers & Fordham 1995:122) although there has been an increase in the number of male carers during the past 10 years. In 1990 the number of people who were recognised as informal carers in the UK was 6.8 million people or 15% of the population (Ackers & Fordham 1995:122, OPCS 1992). This obviously represents a substantial saving for the government, since informal care is clearly a cheaper alternative to formal provision. The range of services provided by informal carers is diverse. These services can include washing clients, assisting clients with walking, taking clients to toilet, cooking, providing company for clients, providing transport, helping clients to talk and advocacy.

Wilmott & Thomas (1984) categorised the tasks as follows:

- Personal care, e.g. washing and toileting
- Domestic care, e.g. cooking, laundering
- Auxiliary care, e.g. shopping, transport

- Social support, e.g. companionship, visiting
- Surveillance, e.g. keeping a watch on elderly people.

Parker & Lawton (1985) classified eight caring activities in the General Household Survey of 1985:

- Help with personal care, e.g. dressing, toileting
- Physical help, e.g. walking
- Help with paperwork and financial matters
- Other practical help, e.g. preparing meals
- Keeping the client company
- Taking the client out
- Giving medication, injections
- Keeping an eye on the client to see that he or she is all right.

Obviously with such an extensive range of possible services, the role of the informal carer is likely to be more time consuming than those of professional carers who will have other clients to attend to. This extensive role is likely to be viewed as an improved form of care since the informal carer knows the client well and, being closely attached to the client, is likely to be very sensitive to his or her needs. However, this attachment may have a cost. Informal carers are not expected to become detached from their clients, yet this detachment is recognised as beneficial to professional carers who are encouraged to 'switch-off' and 'unwind' when their work is completed. Indeed, the stress felt by informal carers is a serious concern which has not gone unnoticed by the government, since the 'Caring for People' White Paper identifies the needs of the carers as well as the clients. Respite care is offered to informal carers who need to take a holiday and unwind. Unfortunately this provision is limited to holiday entitlements and does not allow carers to unwind on a daily or more regular basis. Informal care is likely to lead to less stress on an individual carer if the caring role can be shared between a number of carers, for example a large family or a neighbourhood of willing people able to share out the caring roles and responsibilities. This requires the spirit of neighbourliness as highlighted above. It is rather ironic that for community care to be successful – a desire of the Conservative government, albeit on economic grounds – the spirit of neighbourliness which existed in the immediate post-war years is necessary, yet it is a spirit which appears to have been singularly undermined by the monetarist policies of successive Conservative governments.

Informal care obviously has built-in strengths, since it allows clients a greater independence and choice, but these strengths may be exaggerated. Not all clients wish to live with their relatives, seeing themselves as a burden, particularly if this option means that they must leave their own home and move in with a family member. The clients may further recognise the need for carers to give up their independence, in order to be able to perform the role of informal carer. This may be a sacrifice the clients would not expect or want their family to make. In the 1990s many families depend on dual incomes to survive, and many women work and have careers. This reduces the availability of family members who are able to care for their relatives or forces people to give up their careers, with resultant reduction in family income. Moreover, since the

Case study 11.3	The choice between home and residential care

Derek has lived in a residential home for elderly people for two years since he became disabled following a severe stroke. The stroke left Derek needing help to wash and to dress and to get from his bed to his wheelchair. Although the stroke affected his speech, Derek is still coherent and easy to understand.

Initially, Derek resisted the move to a residential home, preferring to live with one of his children. This was impractical, however, since his elder son, Philip, lived and worked 250 miles away and his daughter June lived locally but in a small three bedroomed semi-detached house with her husband, two children and her mother-in-law (who had lived with them since her husband had died); the younger son, Paul, worked in America. Derek had found it difficult to come to terms with the fact that his three children were not able to care for him in their own home and he had felt rejected. The children had experienced feelings of guilt and felt as if they had let their father down.

After two years of living in the residential home, Derek's views have, however, changed. He accepts that his family were right. The home is excellent and the staff are supportive. Derek is not lonely but feels the staff have helped him to maintain his dignity. He greatly looks forward to seeing his family who visit regularly, and two old friends who still live within the locality also make regular visits to play chess and bridge (two of Derek's lifelong interests) and to take Derek to the nearby bowls club where he is a valued spectator. Derek realises that the decision to enter residential care was a difficult one but readily accepts that his family made the right decision on his behalf.

This case study illustrates the choice between home-based community care or residential care. It shows that in many cases residential care is the only option. It also reveals that even in circumstances where there is no choice, residential care can be excellent and can be an integrated part of community care, not a separate entity.

family model of the 1980s has shifted from the extended to the nuclear, elderly clients are likely to be relocated into a different community in order to live with their relatives, away from their friends, neighbours and familiar surroundings. Obviously this is less than ideal and indicates some of the reasons why informal care can be unsatisfactory.

Residential care can offer some clients a better option. Some clients might prefer to live in a residential home close to their friends and neighbours, where they do not feel a burden on their families (Ackers & Fordham 1995).

Informal care is likely to continue to be an expanding area of social care provision, since the government will continue to support it on economic grounds , but there are nevertheless constraints that will inhibit its expansion. These constraints are:

- geographic, since many prospective carers live away from their invalid relatives because of employment
- gender, since carers of both sexes may need to work
- family type, since nuclear families are less likely to provide informal carers.

Where informal carers do continue to provide services their request for professional support may increase as they become more aware of what is available within the area of statutory support. Requests for assessments under the Carers (Recognition and Services) Act 1995 will increase the workload of care managers and ultimately involve a wide range of professionals and practitioners within the multidisciplinary teams. This will require increased contributions from the NHS, local authorities, housing authorities and education departments.

The requests for respite care are also more likely to increase as carers become more willing to access the facility. The informal sector is likely to develop in sophistication and knowledge as well as in size, and this might place extra requests for resources onto government funding in the future. However, notwithstanding this possibility, the informal sector is always likely to offer governments a cheap alternative of health and social care provision.

The Significance for Nursing

The NHS and Community Care Act (1990) and the Health of the Nation White Paper (DoH 1992) have greatly affected the role of professional people working within the health and social care sector in the 1990s. Members of the nursing profession are likely to have experienced a change in their roles. These might include a shift of emphasis from treatment to prevention, a greater involvement in screening and health promotion or a greater contact with local community. Nurses now are likely to work more closely with an ever-widening range of professionals as greater links are forged between primary and secondary providers and between health and social care providers. With the introduction of the White Paper 'The New NHS: Modern: Dependable' (DoH 1997) the immediate future is likely to continue to be a time of change.

The role of nursing in decision making was increased with the introduction of consensus management in the 1974 reorganisation of the NHS. These measures provided the nursing profession with a direct input into management. This power was very much reduced during the 1980s when the Conservative government favoured a move towards general management and co-opted managers from the world of business. Despite nurses and midwives being the largest component of the employed workforce they were rarely employed as general managers within the new structures of health service management and their direct input in decision making was reduced (Baggott 1994, Glynn & Perkins 1995). These changes were in direct opposition to the proposals of a Green Paper of 1986 entitled 'Neighbourhood nursing: a focus for care' (DHSS 1986) which became known as the 'Cumberledge report'. This report emphasised the need to raise the profile of nurses within the community, giving them more autonomy and responsibility. The suggestion that nurses should prescribe drugs was introduced and the complete autonomy of GPs was challenged by the proposed elevated role of nurses. The proposals received little government support, as they were seen as directly challenging the status of the GPs; this was a political contest the Conservative government did not wish to enter (Baggott 1994:206).

As we have seen, the Conservative government preferred to introduce a mixed economy of care, which essentially increased the importance of GPs as primary care was developed at the expense of secondary care. One reason for this shift in resources was the move towards decentralisation, which the Conservative government favoured, with increased local accountability. Unfortunately clients who were poor were discouraged from accessing the services they genuinely needed, since they were expected to meet the cost of some services, notably prescription charges. The NHS and Community Care Act 1990 invited larger GP practices to apply for fundholding status, giving them even greater autonomy and a budget which allowed them to purchase specific secondary services. This further increased the importance of the primary health-care providers (see Chapter 10). As the primary and community health and care sectors have developed, there has been a move towards integration of the services, and a recognition that the needs of clients treated within their homes are likely to be met by a multidisciplinary team. Nurses are likely to be central players in multidisciplinary work and opportunities to work in the community are likely to expand, since the NHS Act requested that social services departments highlight health problems of local communities and work together with health authorities to meet these needs. The Carers (Recognition and Services) Act 1995 required care managers to co-ordinate packages of support for carers and clients with varied needs, and health services to contribute to multidisciplinary teams to meet them.

Where these opportunities arise the need to develop skill mixes in which all practitioners are thoroughly 'au fait' with their roles and responsibilities is seen as essential. This approach is no longer a new concept as most professionals working within a multidisciplinary structure are devising and developing workable packages. However, there is a need for additional training in which the multidisciplinary approach could be introduced into the initial training of all health and care professions and added to existing curricula.

Working in the community incorporates both curative and preventative models of health care and, with 'Health of the Nation' targets requiring additional resources to be given to areas of prevention and health promotion, nurses are likely to spend a greater part of their work in an advisory and educational capacity. Within the hospital sector, specialist nurses with expertise in a specific illness or disease, e.g. Parkinson's disease, epilepsy or diabetes, are being asked to work within the hospital as well as in the community in an advisory position (see the section 'An Outline of Community Care'; p 235). Future developments may see these nurse specialists given the responsibility of prescribing certain drugs (which interestingly brings us back to the issues raised by the Cumberledge Green Paper).

Closer links between the health authorities and the local authorities are likely to bring closer links between nurses and social workers and social care. The extent of the links is difficult to predict, but the likely result is the expansion of the role of nursing within community social care, as a development of nurses' traditional areas of employment such as employees in nursing homes and as district nurses. The traditional nursing role within hospital wards, casualty departments and operating theatres will not disappear. Clients needing hospital care will still need the services that nurses have always traditionally given, although support workers who are able to acquire competence-based qualifications, such as NVQs, and the Joseph Rowntree Foundation Certificate in Care, are likely to take on much of the traditional work of nursing auxiliaries.

The 'Health of the Nation' targets are likely to strengthen the traditional nursing roles as curative measures and treatment will always be needed, even if sophisticated health promotion and health education packages are developed. The role of nurses may follow that of midwives, many of whom spend periods of time working in the hospital followed by periods of time working in the community. Nursing, as a profession will continue to develop, even though the use of sophisticated computer systems will affect the role of nursing administration, the essentially traditional role that nurses have provided will remain. As Rodwell identifies in his interview of Maureen Raper, a retired health visitor:

> 'young mothers and the elderly will always need face-to-face contact. There is a great future for health visitors because they are professional carers and listeners and they are in contact in the home. So they can, for instance, spot if a mother has post-natal depression. They can refer people on quickly.'
> (Rodwell 1997:23)

The future for all health professionals, including nurses, will almost certainly change as a result of the General Election of 1997. The Labour government is antagonistic to the mixed economy of care, which is seen as providing an unfair service within which opportunities are not the same for all clients. Indeed, the poorer members of society are seen as being disadvantaged further, since they are not able to access private health care. For this reason the Labour government has also suggested that it intends to abolish fundholding in general practice which is seen as providing a two-tier system in which clients of non-fundholding GPs receive a poorer service than clients of fundholders (see Chapter 10).

The 'Mixed Economy of Care' is to be replaced by 'Integrated Care' based on partnership and driven by performance (DoH 1997:5). This is likely to have major consequences on the roles of health professionals. The commitment of the Labour government to primary care suggests that the skill mixes recently developed in GP practices – by, for example, community nurses, health visitors and practice nurses – are areas which will continue to develop.

Indeed, GPs and nurses are expected to take an increasingly influential role in the new NHS. The development of NHS Direct – a 24-hour nurse helpline – is just one example of the increased importance of nursing to the new primary care services. The recognition that local doctors and nurses are the people 'in the best position to know what patients need and hence will be in the driving seat in shaping services' (DoH 1997:11) is a very welcome key principle of the White Paper.

The family doctor and community nurse are recognised as 'the first port of call' for patients seeking health advice and treatment (DoH 1997:32), and the White Paper explains how these groups of professionals will take the lead in developing primary and community health care. Consequently 'Primary Care Groups' will be developed to meet the local needs of patients. These groups should increase the opportunity for nurses to contribute more thoroughly to decision making and hence to the increased quality of primary health care services.

The White Paper's emphasis is on 10-year evolution, not on immediate radical reform. It is hoped that this will give doctors and nurses sufficient time to develop a quality service which is 'there when patients need it' – a central objective of the White Paper. (See Chapter 10 for further discussion of the Labour government's innovations.)

Discussion questions 11.1

The 'mixed economy of care' has given clients within the community a great deal of choice since they can access services from the independent sector as well as the statutory sector. This is undoubtedly a good thing.

Discuss this statement with your peer group. Points to consider may include:

the realities of choice

the costs of individual care packages

the tensions between formal and informal care.

Summary

This chapter has presented an outline of community health and care in the UK in the 1990s. It has not intended to cover all the areas of health and social care which are available within local communities, nor has it been possible to identify all the voluntary agencies which exist within your community. Indeed, an appetite for the community and local provision of health and care services is best satisfied by visiting the locality and meeting some of the providers of the services. The activities within this chapter are intended to help you structure these interests and to find out more about your local community.

The chapter has identified the changes which have occurred in the community since 1990 and the introduction of the Community Care Act. You will be aware now that the services are essentially primary health care and social care and that these two areas are interlinked. The chapter has also attempted to indicate that these links are likely to strengthen in the near future, by the identification of the recommendations of the Carers (Recognition and Services) Act 1995.

The role of the informal care sector has been explored and the difficulties faced by both client and carers within this sector have been analysed. The influence of nursing within the community has also been discussed and the possible changes in the role of nursing in the future have been analysed. These changes are seen as developing and specialisation with a variety of opportunities and areas of work and study. The political need for community care has been examined alongside demographic changes, particularly the increasing elderly population. These changes have forced the government to look for different methods of care provsion.

The expansion of the voluntary sector and particularly the informal sector has given the government a cheaper alternative to statutory provision, and is seen as the major incentive for the development of community care. These developments have not gone uncriticised, and this chapter has attempted to highlight some of the major areas of dissatisfaction.

Further Reading

Baggott R 1994 Health and health care in Britain. Macmillan, London
This is an excellent all round text covering all aspects of health and social care including NHS and community provision.

Billis D, Harris M 1996 Voluntary agencies: challenges of organisation and management. Macmillan, London
This is a useful text for students who wish to explore the voluntary services in more depth.

Local Community Trust. Annual Reports
Within your community you should acquire a copy of the annual reports of your local community trust as these will identify local priorities.

References

Ackers L, Fordham J 1995 Contemporary social policy. The Open Learning Foundation/Churchill Livingstone, Edinburgh

Baggott R 1994 Health and health care in Britain. Macmillan, London

Billis D, Harris M 1996 Voluntary agencies: challenges of organisation and management. Macmillan, London

DHSS 1971 Better services for the mentally handicapped, Cmnd. 4683. HMSO, London

DHSS 1975 Better services for the mentally ill, Cmnd. 6223. HMSO, London

DHSS 1976 Priorities for health and personal social services in England. HMSO, London

DHSS 1986 Neighbourhood nursing: a focus for care (Cumberledge Report). HMSO, London

DoH 1989a Promoting better health. HMSO, London

DoH 1989b Working for patients, Cmnd. 555. HMSO, London

DoH 1989c Caring for people, Cmnd. 849. HMSO, London

DoH 1991 The Patients' Charter. HMSO, London

DoH 1992 The health of the nation. HMSO, London

DoH 1995 The Carers (Recognition and Services) Act. HMSO, London

DoH 1996a The Carers (Recognition and Services) Act 1995: policy guidance. DoH, London

DoH 1996b The Carers (Recognition and Services) Act 1995: practice guide. DoH, London

DoH 1997 The new NHS: Modern: Dependable. Cmnd. 3807. HMSO, London

Glynn JJ, Perkins DA 1995 Managing health care: challenges for the 90's. WB Saunders, London

Griffiths R 1988 Community care: agenda for action. HMSO, London

Ham C 1992 Health policy in Britain: the politics and organisation of the National Health Service, 3rd edn. Macmillan, London

Labour Party 1997 General election manifesto. Labour Party, London

MacErlean N 1997 Money matters: thrown off the ward and into the wild. The Observer, 14 September:22

Meredith B 1993 The community care handbook: the new system explained. Age Concern, London

OPCS 1992 General household survey 1990. GHS22. HMSO, London

Parker G, Lawton D cited in OPCS 1992 General Household Survey 1990. GHS22. HMSO, London

Rodwell L 1997 NHS Magazine, Issue 10, Autumn 1997. NHS Executive, London

Thatcher M 1993 The Downing Street Years. HarperCollins, London

Wilmott P, Thomas D 1984 Community in social policy. Policy Studies Institute, London

SOCIOLOGICAL PERSPECTIVES IN NURSING

Key concepts

- Changing roles in nursing
- Nursing practice
- Nursing and social theories
- The importance of being a nurse
- Weaving the strands together

The final and concluding section synthesises much of what has preceded and promotes understanding of the significance of the theoretical perspectives of sociology to nursing. The changing role of women in society and the corresponding impact on nursing roles make interesting and perhaps controversial reading as the feminist movement in nursing and midwifery is highlighted.

In concluding, Section 5 encourages the development of a personal perspective which can form the basis for positive reflective practice based in knowledge gained through introspection informed by sociological knowledge, nursing theory and personal practice.

12 Nursing and Social Theory

Mary Birchenall and Peter Birchenall

Key concepts	■ Changing roles in nursing
	■ Nursing practice
	■ Nursing and social theories
	■ The importance of being a nurse
	■ Weaving the strands together

We now begin to tie together some of the wider issues evident in the social world that impinge on the nurse and nursing. This chapter has as its central focus the influence of sociological understandings on nursing work and nursing theory. We will begin with the role of the nurse, move on to the practice of nursing and so to an elucidation of some of the underpinning sociology that informs theories of nursing.

Changing Roles in Nursing

Nursing developed from the modest beginnings of heroic figures such as Florence Nightingale whose energies focused on the 'doing' of work. Modern gurus of 'doing', such as Benner, elaborate the work of the nurse in complex theoretical formulations that seem set to contribute to the two tiers suggested by Fatchett (1994) who, reflecting on recent changes in nursing, writes about the possible, and perhaps now more likely,

> 'creation of a two-tier system of health carers. One tier will be made up of an elite minority of well-paid nurse professionals who will manage and organize care, and the other, lesser tier will be made of non-professional carers who will carry out the prescribed tasks needed to keep the NHS in business.'
>
> (Fatchett 1994:118)

Perhaps the need to remove the image of nursing away from those evident in such epic films as the 'Carry On . . .' series has contributed to this idea of a two-tiered nursing service. Public images of nursing retain the notion of the 'angel', the essential helper in times of need and distress. Perhaps rightly, nursing seeks to replace such images with those of a professional person. In turn, it is important to ensure that the positive public image of nursing remains as part of that professional person. Caution is necessary to ensure that the caring images of the nurse, far from being eroded, become the mantle given to the 'lesser non-professional tier' described by Fatchett above.

The image of expert manager of nursing could lead to confusion as to the purpose of such an expensive individual if the required hands-on aspect of care is delivered in a more economical and seemingly more humanistic fashion by an unqualified non-nurse. Caplan (1977), writing about the 'disabling professions', suggested that 'the main difference between a lawyer and a tin of peas is that we do not always know when and whether we need one. . . .' (pp 96–97). This cryptic aspersion of an esteemed profession of long tradition provides a timely caution for nursing in this period of change.

At times it seems that, through the processes of reflection, nursing climbs a steep hill seeking to emerge into the limelight of professionalism. Care must be taken to avoid eradicating on route many human traits necessary to nursing practice. Personal traits such us prejudice are combated daily by nurses. Earlier chapters in this book have considered the consequences of labelling and stigma both for nurses and those for whom they provide care services. Social ills that are still recognised as Beveridge's five evils of 'want', 'ignorance', 'idleness', 'squalor' and 'disease', continue to challenge the nurse and influence the nature of health, despite the passing of more than 50 years since their eradication was promised.

Pearson (1992) writes: 'Nursing, as a collective, frequently misses the point of its very existence: the provision of a nursing service to those who need, seek, or are directed to, nursing.' (Pearson 1992:213). Slavish following of politically determined changes to nursing that enhance professional status but overlook the real consequences for the individual patient or client may have unforeseen implications for the future of nursing. Issues worthy of reflection at this point are the re-creation of tiers of nursing and a refocusing of nursing knowledge towards primary care and health while retaining a service emphasis on illness.

New divisions in nursing that create an elite are far from new. In the late 1960s the creation of the enrolled nurse provided just such a situation. Since the early 1990s the eradication of this tier has been actively promoted as such divisions were unattractive to the development of the professional status of nursing. The move towards advanced educational standing for nurses promises further divisions which may be the harbingers of the future split between professional nursing and hands-on care. These changes in the structure of nursing are evidence of the rift between theory and practice. As nursing theorists seek to elucidate the knowledge of nursing, its practice is being overwhelmed by politicians and the pragmatics of economics. The chapters on the professional aspects of nursing and changes in the structure of care provide some background to this discussion. Additionally, recent emphasis on community health and population studies are likely to promote further changes in the nature of nursing work and the role of the nurse.

Nursing Practice: Community

Politically determined changes have been precipitated into the world of nursing with some rapidity over the last decade. Roper et al (1996), conscious of many developments in nursing practice, are concerned with the ways in which nursing is managing change. They are particularly interested in the mechanisms introduced by nurses to implement the move towards 'Putting Patients First', prompted by politically led changes to the NHS. They see the evolution of primary nursing as providing the pivot for achieving the goal of patient-centred care. These latter theorists identify a nursing strategy to achieve a political imperative that is prompted by a particular social context. Such ideas are reinforced by the recognition that holistic nursing is the emergent paradigm which is likely to become more prominent in the twenty-first century. As such this book has been concerned with the social environment of nursing, ideas concerning the patient/client, and theories about health and illness.

The movements towards community care and health promotion are embraced by nursing. These latter developments are intrinsically linked to the transition from cure to care as the impetus for nursing work; such a movement is greeted with approbation. Yet there seems scope here for a short warning that such changes in the nature of nursing work do not occur in isolation. Indeed, the radical change that centres on the emphasis on health rather than illness carries with it echoes from other social and political changes. The process of change is central to the work of thinkers such as Foucault and has a growing influence on the sociology of medicine and health (Armstrong 1987, Gastaldo 1997, Nettleton & Bunton 1995).

Caring and Gender

Meleis (1987) demands that nursing should develop 'gender sensitive knowledge' and become attuned to global issues and approaches. That

Reflection point 12.1

The following quote provides an insight into the all-pervasive nature of modern health care. You may find it useful to debate the argument set out by Gastaldo using (1) material gleaned from previous readings throughout this book, (2) awareness of changes in your local health-care arena and (3) current discussions in the media.

Gastaldo (1997:116) writes:

'Anatamo-politics ... focuses on the body as a machine (Foucault 1990:139). Docility and usefulness are identified by Foucault as ways to integrate the body into economic and social life. In order to achieve this, the operation of disciplinary power pervades relations in families, schools, hospitals, work, etc. In the case of medicine, the effect of discipline is for the therapeutic space to become a political space. Individuality has been constructed based on symptoms, disease, or lifestyle; control over these processes is at the core of medical care (Foucault 1991:144). The political space that health care and policy constitute is an important site for the exercise of disciplinary power. Focusing on individual bodies or on the social body, health professionals are entitled by scientific knowledge/power to examine, interview and prescribe "healthy" lifestyles.'

Consider the ways in which political decisions have directly influenced and changed the delivery of care to. Focus on the needs of:

people with a learning disability

people with enduring mental illness

the frail older adult.

need remains evident and can be advanced through understanding the nature of the underpinning sociological knowledge embedded in much nursing theory. The influence of feminist theories on health and health care is evident in both nursing and patient worlds. In nursing there is evidence of a 'glass ceiling' that limits the career progression for female nurses and promotes a disproportionate number of men into senior positions. The rights of patients to state preferences as to the gender of their carer are recognised.

'The woman's movement has caused female patients/clients to seek more responsibility for and control over their bodies, health, and lives in general. As women become more aware of their own needs and unique qualities, they seek health care that can help them meet those needs.'
(Heath 1995:15)

As with any social movement the demands by women to redress centuries of inequalities has been countered by a 'backlash', and the rights of men have a growing focus in health care. There is a growing incidence of 'well-men clinics' and recognition that the emotional needs of men are legitimate and need acknowledgement.

Nursing and Social Theories

The uncritical assumption of theory and then a naive application through the theoretical formulations of nursing can be problematic. It is essential that any new ideas, however enticing, are understood within their originating context before they become deified within nursing. The impact of the theory of 'normalisation' on services for people with a learning disability and its more general penetration into the realms of primary health care will serve to elucidate this latter statement. For a brief overview of normalisation see Chapter 9. Fulcher (1996) writes:

> 'While the normalisation project appeared to be radical, its assumptions were functionalist and its ideas and concerns interactionist (Chappell 1992, Oliver 1994). Such a project left untouched fundamental practices such as the professional control of services (Oliver 1994). Thus despite its apparent radicalism, the normalisation project could be relatively easily inserted into policy statements and practices.'
> (Fulcher 1996:168)

Fulcher adds that normalisation as a functionalist theory is oppressive 'to all but the dominant class'. Ideas of normalisation have become part of the common currency of health language and have certainly permeated the field of learning disability nursing. A perhaps naive interpretation of normalisation theory has resulted in key theorists either rejecting the word (Wolfensberger 1983) or publishing warnings with reference to misconceptions about the term normalisation (Perrin & Nirje 1985). Essentially, people whose lives are directly affected by disability have grave misgivings about a theory viewed by professionals as having the potential to advance care practices and change social values. The links between politics, policy and practice promote a tension between the impact and the philosophical underpinnings of an idea.

Normalisation has evolved as a practice imperative within a social context that recognises the devastating impact of the asylum, the emergence of 'community care' and the development of holism and individualised care practices, while simultaneously evolving a market style economy of care. Additionally, over the last two decades the culture of British society has changed. There is a move away from dependence on the state towards individual independence that is tempered by individual rights and responsibilities to work within normative social behaviours. To this end the family is idealised and regarded as a resource within the political economy of care. Perhaps the current development that urges a 'partnership' between carer and client is evidence of yet another political gloss that disguises a real reduction in services available to those in need. This is particularly evident for those clients with chronic care needs who frequently fall between the health and social definitions of service. The rhetoric of 'partnership' is in sharing, but notions of equal sharing do not seem to be at the fore. The balance between professional and client has always been uneven with the balance being on the side of the knowledgeable professional. Nursing must consider carefully the dilemmas of professionalism with its concomitant promotion for nurses but potential for devaluing the significance of the many basic care aspects of nursing practice.

Nursing as a social entity has evolved in parallel with the above changes, absorbing these realities and changing styles and images perhaps too readily and without taking time for an analysis of the impact of change. The reluctance of political agendas to combat the effects of material deprivation take on a new dimension when viewed in conjunction with the emergence of health education. The individual, not medicine, has become the key to good health, and as such contributes to the dissonant developments between theory and practice. There should be no surprises then that a theory such as that of 'normalisation' should permeate the layers of health care and begin to widely influence nursing practice. Normalisation centres on retaining the key functions of the dominant sectors of society and emphasises the deviancy substructures of disability and illness, despite the apparent emphasis on normal lifestyles and empowerment. In this way a seemingly positive theory can be manipulated to maintain the status quo, and further delineate the division between carer and cared for, rather than contributing to the acceptance of difference as a social norm. Nursing, therefore, needs to consider carefully the origins of any theory that promotes change. A balance is needed between resistance and uptake that encourages reflection at the professional as well as the personal level.

The Importance of Being a Nurse

The feminist sociologist, Ann Oakley, wrote in 1993 a book entitled 'Essays on Women, Medicine and Health'. Chapter 4 of this book is entitled 'On the importance of being a nurse' and is concerned with her account of what she considers to be the significant factors in the work of nursing that create a potentially unique role. She reminds us that nursing was concerned with care when medicine was firmly rooted in cure. In tracing the history of nursing Oakley highlights the nuances of difference between the 'professional' elite of medicine and law and the professionalisation of nursing. This impetus towards the recognition of the professional nature of nursing need not remove the essential skills of nursing that are embedded in notions of care. The strongly masculine aspects of the feminist movement in nursing perhaps need tempering with feminine strengths. These strengths are at the centre of caring and they need recognition within the nursing profession before the masculinisation of nursing can remove what is an inherent strength. Writing about developments in consumer power Oakley is concerned that, if nursing aligns with the professional elite, then the links with the emotional needs of patients will be minimised.

> 'When we look at surveys of how patients feel about nurses the importance of caring emerges very clearly. People prefer nurses to be warm, kind, sympathetic personalities. . . . On the theme of emotional support, one study by Rose Coser in the USA found that patients see the nurse's essential task as giving personal reassurance and emotional support. . . . Caring about, and for, the patient is therefore an important part of the nurse's role in practice – whatever the theory.'
> (Oakley 1993:46–47)

On the theme of professionalisation and the links between theory and practice, it is apparent that nursing could suffer a damaged reputation. The potential creation of elite groups as a consequence of changing educational and political climates may be a force that weakens rather than strengthens nursing if the underlying theories that drive such change remain unexamined. Perhaps nursing should question the superiority of professional status; after all professionalisation may well damage the nation's health.

Social theory then can be seen as inextricably linked to the practice of nursing. The defining of the patient, and the determination of treatment and care are influenced at some point by social interpretations of the situation. Fundamental to the individual, whether nurse or patient, are the processes of primary and secondary socialisation, through which the individual orders his or her personal social world. Nurses as social beings are subject to social pressures which influence their practice and understandings of their role. Fundamental decisions that appear deliberate to the individual can originate through unconscious influences. Nurses, in ordering their professional lives, need to be overtly aware of the nature of the social world in which they practice. This awareness requires that taken-for-granted assumptions, about such notions as 'class', 'gender', 'wealth' and others that have featured in the chapters of this book are recognised as part of an examinable social world.

Reflection point 12.2

Oakley (1993) suggests the following key issues that are significant for modern nursing. They provide an interesting range of ideas that nursing needs to debate.

You may like to consider exploring these issues through the literature and from your experiences in practice.

- Nursing emerged in the mid-nineteenth century as a specialised form of domestic work.
- A major constraint in the development of nursing is the gender division of labour in health care.
- Nurses should reshape their place in health care to ally more closely with needs of patients. They should avoid becoming oppressive professionals.
- Caring and emotional support are the core aspects of the nursing role.
- The experience of nursing is that caring is important, but the dominant culture denies this, dismissing caring as of low value. Such values threaten the integrity of nursing and may force an assumption of masculine values that will remove the special skills of nursing.

Weaving the Strands Together

Emerging themes from the book bind together to form a matrix of understanding about the place of sociology and social policy in health care. An exploration of these themes has illustrated how health as a concept is inextricably linked to lifestyle and the quality of the social environment within which people exist. Social institutions such as the family make complex demands on a health service that is pledged to care for each of us as we progress through life. As human beings we are uniquely different from each other and these differences reflect who we are, our perceived place in the social order, our attitudes to personal health and the way we respond to external influences on our health status. These influences include government campaigns to reduce deaths from smoking-related disease, alcohol and other drug abuse, coronary artery disease and poverty.

Our awareness of social issues and health continues to increase, particularly through research evidence that links poverty, poor housing and unemployment with ill-health and premature death. Despite the existence of a health service that purports to be free at the point of delivery and a welfare state that seeks to support people in social need, there remain sections of the population that fall through the net. For example, homeless people as a group face risks to their health because of exposure to inclement weather and poor diet. Travelling people have health needs that are neglected principally because of a lifestyle that constantly moves them from place to place with a consequence that they do not comply with the official health-care expectation that they register with a general practitioner.

We have explored gender, ethnicity, the ageing population and citizenship in relation to the provision of health care and we recognise that certain well-established attitudes and practices still exist where various social groups experience forms of discrimination in the way their medical needs are diagnosed and treated. It is in relation to this that nurses should reflect on their own attitudes towards these and other groups, particularly people that attract a specific label through demonstrating mental health problems, severe learning disability or through just being old, frail or incontinent. Reinforcement of a negative label is often at the heart of a client or patient becoming unpopular with nursing staff and we have seen how difficult it can be to remove the stigma associated with labelling. By virtue of their role in society, nurses are held in esteem by the general population and as such are in a unique relationship position with their patients/clients. We have seen how this relationship, and the power base that it creates, can work against the best interests of those being cared for. In particular we examined how nursing care, as currently conceived, can effectively disempower patients and clients despite the official desire to increase their independence. Complaining is often done out of the earshot of nurses and we looked at research carried out on a surgical ward that suggested such behaviour may be useful for relieving tension and frustration. It forms part of the social support network that hospitalised patients provide for each other. The nurse is viewed as a gatekeeper for other health-care professions, particularly medical staff. The nurse guards information from the patients/clients and relatives which in itself gives nurses power and control over people's lives.

The realities of nursing as a profession, and the relationship between the nurse and other professionals, is changing, and we had explored some of these changes. There is still some confusion as to whether nursing fits the template of professional status. This debate, although somewhat circular, will continue and interesting times lie ahead when nursing is asked to embrace occupational standards and take account of such issues as National Vocational Qualifications when deciding what to accept as the qualifying standard for becoming a Registered Nurse. Thorny issues surrounding the development of generic nursing will remain on the agenda just as will the move towards an all-graduate profession and the increasing influence of higher education on nursing curricula. The marketplace of caring is dynamic, and social and economic policy will make demands on nursing to change direction on a regular basis. The days of 'permanent change' are with us and nursing will have to refocus regularly in the face of current market forces and the mixed economy of care; this applies to both statutory and independent health providers.

Summary　This concluding chapter has considered some perspectives that will help in developing further the sociological interpretation of nursing and nursing work. Medicine and illness beliefs have polarised in professional terms between the notions of 'cure' and 'care'. More specifically, in nursing, interpretations of the functions of the nurse in health care provide a further dichotomy: that of doctor's handmaiden or professional. As the theory that underpins nursing work emerges in more concrete ways, the extensive demands that holistic care practices make on the individual practitioner become overt. This book has pursued the social dimensions of health, illness and nursing work. In so doing the complexity of nursing work becomes evident. The social context of nursing and the social world of the nurse are part of the foundations for holistic care.

Discussion questions 12.1

- How may the status of 'professional' change the work of the nurse?
- Consider the role of the informal carer in relation to the professional nurse and reflect on the extent to which imbalances in power may impair the relationship.
- To what extent do you and your peers consider the tensions of gender and 'race' to be significant to nursing and nursing practice?

Further Reading

Fatchett A 1994 Politics policy and nursing. Baillière Tindall, London

This book provides a critical review of the impact of changes in the NHS on the delivery of health services and some consequences for nursing work. It is an interesting read.

Scambler G (ed) 1991 Sociology as applied to medicine, 3rd edn. Baillière Tindall, London

This book advances many of the arguments explored here. It is somewhat more dense in its style than this book but is useful for the individual reader who wishes to go beyond the introductory review offered in this book.

Bornat J et al (eds) 1993 Community care: a reader. The Open University, Milton Keynes

This book provides a review of community care policy and practice issues relevant to all branches of nursing.

Walmsley J et al (eds) 1993 Health welfare and practice reflecting on roles and relationships. Sage Publications in association with the Open University, London

This book provides a range of discussions on the nature of professioanl roles, and the links to empowerment and power. The final section reflects on the implications of professional roles for practice. This is a highly readable book.

References

Armstrong D 1987 Bodies of knowledge: Foucault and the problem of human anatomy. In: Scambler G (ed) Sociological theory and medical sociology. Tavistock Publications, London, Ch 3

Caplan J 1977 Lawyers and litigants: a cult reviewed. In: Illich I et al (eds) Disabling professions. Marion Boyars, London, New York

Chappell A L 1992 Towards a sociological critique of the normalisation principle. Disability and Society 9(2): 123–144

Fatchett A 1994 Politics policy and nursing. Baillière Tindall, London

Foucault M 1990 The history of sexuality, vol. 1: an introduction. Penguin, London

Foucault M 1991 Discipline and punish: the birth of the prison. Penguin, London

Fulcher G 1996 Beyond normalisation but not Utopia. In: Barton L (ed) Disability and society: emerging issues and insights. Longman, London, Ch 9

Gastaldo D 1997 Is health education good for you? Re-thinking health education through the concept of bio-power. In: Peterson A, Bunton R (eds) Foucault, health and medicine. Routledge, London, Ch 6

Heath HBM (ed) 1995 Potter and Perry's foundations in nursing theory and practice. Mosby, St Louis

Meleis A 1987 Revisions in knowledge development: a passion for substance. Scholarly Enquiry for Nursing Practice: An International Journal 1(1): 5–19

Nettleton S, Bunton R 1995 Sociological critiques of health promotion. In: Bunton R, Nettleton S, Burrows R (eds) The sociology of health promotion critical analyses of consumption lifestyle and risk. Routledge, London, Ch 4

Oakley A 1993 Essays on women, medicine and health. Edinburgh University Press, Edinburgh

Oliver M 1994 Capitalism, disability and ideology: a materialist critique of the normalization principle. Paper presented at an international conference on normalization at the University of Ottawa, Canada

Pearson A 1992 Knowing nursing: emerging paradigms in nursing. In: Robinson K, Vaughan B (eds) Knowledge for nursing practice. Butterworth Heinemann, Oxford, London, Ch 14

Perrin B, Nirje B 1985 Setting the record straight: a critique of some frequent misconceptions of the normalization principle. Australian and New Zealand Journal of Developmental Disabilities

Roper N, Logan WW, Tierney AJ 1996 The elements of nursing: a model for nursing based on a model of living, 4th edn. Churchill Livingstone, Edinburgh

Wolfensberger W 1983 Social role valorisation: a proposed new term for the principle of normalization. Mental Retardation 21(8): 234–239

Glossary

Ageism Prejudicial actions based on age usually towards the older adult.

Alternative therapies A range of therapies (usually provided within the private sector) which include non-traditional health-care treatment, e.g. acupuncture, hypnosis, etc.

Artefact A manufactured or man-made compilation of factors or statistics.

Class Social divisions evident in British society.

Community A locality or small area where people share common interests.

Compliance Unquestioned agreement with a medical decision affecting one's personal health status.

Consumer sovereignty The respect for individual choice in a range of services from education to health care.

Contract Formal agreement between a provider of health services and a purchaser.

Credentialism In education: a process whereby individuals are measured according to their success in gaining recognised qualifications.

Demographic changes Changes which occur within a population, e.g. unemployment statistics.

Deviance (primary) Social rule breaking that has little or no effect on the person's other social roles.

Deviance (secondary) Social rule breaking that has a profound effect on the person's other social roles.

Disability A term used to define those who are considered as having physical or intellectual abilities that are less than the norm.

Discrimination Activities and behaviour towards others resulting from prejudicial values.

Emotional labour The usually 'hidden' work relating to the management of feelings which health workers carry out in order for health goals to be met. Mostly performed by low-status workers.

Ethnomethodology The study of ordinary people's methods for making sense of, and creating order in, everyday life.

Family The grouping of individuals who are related to each other through ties of blood, marriage or adoption. Traditionally the family is viewed as an economic unit responsible for the nurturing and upbringing of children.

Feminism Defining the explicit presence of women in the social world and their equality to men in all spheres of life.

Formal caring   Care provided by official agencies, inclusive of charitable foundations; usually delivered by paid workers.

Functionalism   A significant perspective in sociology which is concerned with the structures and functions of society.

Fundholding General Practitioner (FHGP)   A GP who receives a budget from the RHA to control the practice. Fundholders provide primary health care and purchase secondary health care.

Gender   A distinguishing status (male or female) applied to the biological sex.

Health   The World Health Organization defines health as being more than the absence of disease. Health is a physical and emotional status that is influenced by environmental and societal factors.

Humiliation   The feeling experienced by many clients on first encountering many health-care situations, e.g. the lack of privacy, which creates the vulnerability and imbalance of status which disempowers clients.

Independent sector   The combined care services of the private and voluntary sectors: they are deemed to be independent of the public sectors (NHS and DSS).

Informal caring   Care provided without formal organisation; usually provided by friends, family members or neighbours.

Interpretivism   Interpretation of the social world by social actors.

Labelling   The ascribing of a negative label to an action that is then taken up as a means of defining the person. Also called **social judgement**.

Meritocracy   A system in which ability is rewarded and success gains merit.

Minority ethnic group   Groups of people who share a culture that is markedly different from the dominant group in any particular society.

Mixed economy of care   Open market of health and social care in which providers of statutory sector and independent sector compete for contracts.

Multi-agency care   Care in which separate professional agencies co-operate to provide client-focused care.

Normalisation   Promoting a shared set of values and beliefs that form the fabric of a civilised society enabling people to fit in and feel comfortable in their social role.

Poverty   Exclusion from the benefits and advantages which are considered normal for most people in society; living on the margins of society without power or public voice to express concerns.

Poverty (absolute)   Insufficient material benefits to maintain life.

Poverty (relative)   Life experiences below the material standards normal for that society.

Prejudice   Negative attitudes and values directed towards specific groups of people or individuals.

Private health sector   Providers of health and care services that are profit making and charge for services.

Professions   Occupations demonstrating commonality of particular ideologies and institutional traits.

'Race'   A term resting on the assumption that human beings are divided into different groups as a result of biological properties.

Sentimental work   Analogous to **emotional labour**.

Social actors   People who make up the world and the roles they occupy.

Social control   The mechanisms evident to ensure social order.

Social institution   A way of referring to particular social groupings that are common to the majority of people in society.

Social judgement   See **labelling**

Social mobility   The movement upwards or downwards between social classes.

Social policy   Decisions made at government level that determine the quality of health and social care locally.

Social stratification   Divisions within society of which social class is one; it extends to include also other layers such as gender and race.

Sociology   The study of human life ranging from the individual to groups and societies.

Sociological theory   An exploration of the relationships between different areas and kinds of social life; it involves classifying and understanding the conditions under which certain processes and patterns of structure or conflict are likely to occur in society.

Statutory sector   Sector established by law; clients can access services as legal right, e.g. personal social services, NHS.

Stigma   The consequences of a negative label applied to an individual.

Structuralism   A term used to describe and understand the construction and maintenance of societies.

Symbolic interactionism   A sociological perspective that uses the structures of language to explore meaning.

Total institution   An institution cut off from the rest of the social world in which inmates work, rest and play in the same place.

Trust hospital   Self-governing provider of secondary health care.

Vocationalism   A selfless dedicated form of work centred around the patient or client.

Voluntary sector   Non-profit-making organisations, including charitable organisations, e.g. Age Concern, Mind.

Index

Page numbers in italics refer to boxed material